AROMATHERAPY FOR WOMEN

How to use the subtle powers of essential oils to enhance
every aspect of a woman's life.

AROMATHERAPY
FOR WOMEN
Beautifying and Healing Essences
from Flowers and Herbs

by

MAGGIE TISSERAND

THORSONS PUBLISHING GROUP

First published April 1985

© MAGGIE TISSERAND 1985

Illustrated by Paul Turner

British Library Cataloguing in Publication Data

Tisserand, Maggie
Aromatherapy for women.
1. Essences and essential oils. – Therapeutic use
I. Title
615'.32   RM666.A68

ISBN 0-7225-1119-1

Published by Thorsons Publishers Limited,
Wellingborough, Northamptonshire, NN8 2RQ, England.

Printed in Great Britain by Richard Clay Limited,
Bungay, Suffolk.

9   11   13   15   14   12   10

DEDICATION

To women everywhere and all they care for.

CONTENTS

Page

Introduction   9

Chapter
1. Getting Through the Day   13
2. Gynaecological Remedies   29
3. Sexuality and Sensuality   35
4. Health and Healing   45
5. Skin and Hair Care   63
6. Pregnancy and Childbirth   75
7. After the Birth   85
8. Remedies for Childhood Illnesses   91
9. Recipes   107
   Glossary of Methods of Treatment   119
   Further Reading   123
   Useful Addresses   125
   Index   127

INTRODUCTION

This book has been written because, although there are a number of excellent books available on aromatherapy, I wanted to present the subject in simple terms, with the accent on using the essences at home, to alleviate minor health problems, enhance sensuality, and improve upon the appearance of skin and hair.

I am not a therapist, and can claim no qualifications except that I have 'lived and breathed' essential oils ever since marrying Robert Tisserand in 1973, and have accrued a great deal of knowledge in the use of essential oils for health problems, as well as for all my beauty needs.

Robert is viewed by many as being the leading authority on the subject of aromatherapy, and his book *The Art of Aromatherapy* (see Further Reading) is used by aromatherapists all over the world, and by those teaching the subject.

I have drawn largely on my experiences during pregnancy, childbirth and in bringing up three children and the very tangible improvements in my appearance and general state of health, but also on feedback from friends and relatives who have benefited from using essential oils. If you are neither pregnant, nor have any young children, then Chapters 6, 7 and 8 may not interest you. But I hope that you will find something in the book which will benefit you in a real way.

In a nutshell, aromatherapy means 'a therapy using aromas'. The aromas come from the plant kingdom – flowers, trees, herbs and bushes. The relevant part of the plant (the wood of the sandalwood tree; the petals from roses; rind from lemon and bergamot fruits; leaves from rosemary bushes) is put through a process known as *distillation*, where the volatile, odiferous substance, is captured. It is this liquid which is known as an *essential oil*. Essential oils (sometimes referred to in this book as *essences*) are highly concentrated, and should always be diluted before being applied to the skin. There are many ways in which essential oils can be used – a few drops on a tissue, for *inhaling*; in vegetable oils, for use as *a massage oil*; a few drops added to the water to create an *aromatic bath*; or simply worn as a *perfume*; but it should always be remembered that essential oils are quite strong and only small amounts are necessary.

The essences, with the exception of the citrus oils, are very long lasting, and provided that they are stored in dark bottles, away from direct sunlight, will last for many years without losing their therapeutic powers. They have the properties of the herb or flower from which they came, but have the advantage of being infinitely more convenient to use.

The term *aromatherapy* was coined in the 1920s to describe the usage of essential oils for therapeutic purposes, but it could just as easily have been called *essential oil therapy* or *plant essence therapy*. I say this, having spoken to people who were confused by the use of the word 'aroma' imagining that the extent of aromatherapy was merely to inhale vapours from a bowl.

Essential oils have many uses, although our sense of smell, being linked to our emotions, plays the largest part in recognizing the power of aromatherapy and here we can discover how certain essences have the power to lift depression, or which essences have a calming influence on troubled emotions when we are under stress. My knowledge of this subject has been the best investment (in terms of health and beauty) that I have ever made, and I hope that by sharing my experience with you, opinionated as it may seem, that you will also find in aromatherapy, a valuable adjunct to other forms of alternative medicine and a very practical, highly enjoyable way of feeling and looking good.

Note:
I do not recommend that the reader try to treat serious or complicated disorders, but should instead seek the help of a qualified aromatherapist or other practitioner.

1.
GETTING THROUGH
THE DAY

During the course of the day, a great many different situations will present themselves to us, and although some of them may be a pleasurable experience, others may be physically demanding or emotionally taxing. This is when **aromatherapy** can help us through the day.

An early morning bath to wake you up

Perhaps, for the third night in succession, one of your children has climbed into your bed and wriggled about for the next few hours, until the alarm clock has released you from the torture. Or your neighbours have held yet another noisy all night party, or your partner's snores constantly beckon you from the dream world. Come morning, you know you can't go back to sleep because you have work to do, or children to take to school, but you don't know how you are going to manage. Your head feels dull and aches, you feel lethargic and irritable. I felt this way on the morning of my driving test, because my youngest daughter had yet again crept in during the night. I needed a strong stimulant, so I had a **rosemary** bath. It stimulates the nervous system and clears the head very quickly. Just a ten to fifteen minute bath is long enough to feel the benefits, although there is no maximum length of time. As usual,

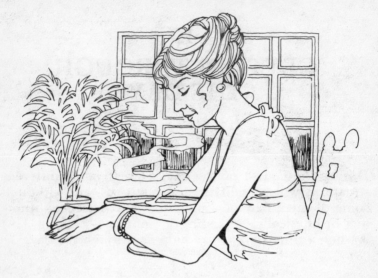

my rosemary bath left me feeling wide awake and very
alert. If you don't even have time for a bath, just put two
drops of rosemary and two drops of clary sage into a basin
full of hot water. Lean over and inhale the vapours for a
few minutes. I was also feeling nervous on this occasion,
and so I took a drop of **rose** oil in honey water, which is
calming and soothing to fraught nerves. I remember
driving around the Oxfordshire countryside with my test
inspector, in the middle of a storm, complete with
thunder and lightning. But I felt totally confident, calm
and in complete control of myself and the situation, and
needless to say, I passed my test.

Mental Fatigue

Basil oil stimulates the brain and is fantastic to refresh

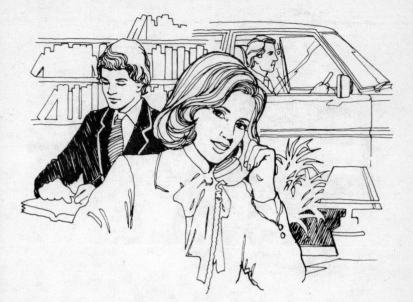

your mental powers during a demanding day in the office, or during examination 'swotting'. It is also ideal for long distance drivers, and generally anyone who has to concentrate for long periods of time, and may consequently suffer from mental fatigue. Because oil of basil is so strong, simply smelling the vapour of just a drop or two on a tissue is sufficient to refresh the grey matter. At times I have been extremely grateful that I have had a bottle of basil in the glove compartment of my car, when driving home on the motorway, and all but dropping off to sleep. For me, basil works even better than a cup of black coffee, and is more convenient, since it is not necessary to first find a motorway cafe. I also keep a bottle of basil oil in my desk drawer, and have an occasional whiff from it on those days when I am mentally below par, and would much rather go to the cinema, but have to stay at my desk.

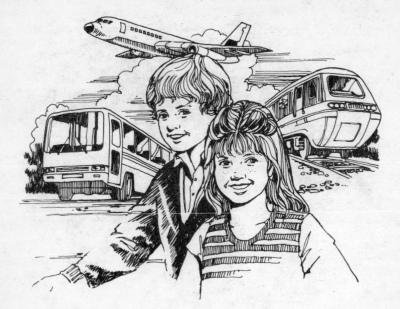

Travel Sickness

When travelling with my children, I always take a bottle of **peppermint** oil and **lavender** oil. Whether flying, sailing or driving, my eldest daughter invariably announces that she feels sick. If she has eaten recently, I let her smell the peppermint oil, as it is renowned for its stomachic properties (calming the stomach). But if she is over-excited about going somewhere new or unfamiliar, then I give her lavender to smell. Lavender is a very calming and soothing essence, and has many uses when travelling. So far, I have never had to stop the car to clean up.

Small children should not be given a bottle to smell in case they spill it, so give them a drop of the chosen essence on a tissue.

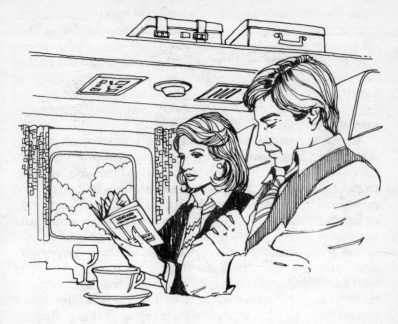

Jet lag

Jet lag is a modern phrase used to describe the way international air travellers feel after long hours in the sky. Symptoms include chronic tiredness, (complete with insomnia); constipation; swollen feet and ankles; confusion; and depression. Some people suffer more acutely than others, and may have to retire to bed for two days. Others are little affected. But it seems impossible to avoid some symptoms of jet lag, as we are forcing our bodies to accept very unnatural conditions – travelling at high speeds, sitting still for eight hours or more, and eating more frequently than we would normally do (to relieve boredom). However, on reaching our destination, a bath with **ylang-ylang** and **lavender** will ensure a relaxed, restful sleep. If your arrival is shortly before a business meeting, etc., then rather than take a cat-nap, have a bath to which you have added **rosemary** and **lemongrass**. This will give you a fresh, energized feeling, and should see you through the rest of the day. The relaxing, night-time bath can be repeated every night, and the revitalizing day-time bath can be used every morning, until your body has adjusted to the changes in time and climate.

There are other ways to avoid a bad case of jet lag. Alcohol causes dehydration, so its consumption is likely to contribute to headaches, constipation and swollen feet. On long flights, I never drink alcohol or coffee, but prefer to drink mineral water to which I add a drop or two of **Rescue Remedy***. I also only eat when I am hungry, and not every time a steward brings around a snack.

Take-off and landing is very traumatic for some people, and I suspect that the fear causes a lot more tension, as well as releasing adrenalin (the well-known flight or fight response). The stress caused to the body under these conditions can be quite considerable. Taking **Rescue Remedy** in water before leaving the airport, and again as soon as drinks are served after take-off, will help even the most nervous travellers to stay calm. Another uplifting tip is to have a tissue impregnated with **clary sage** oil, in a bag or pocket. It will make you feel better, and probably everyone around you as well.

* One of the Bach Flower Remedies (see Further Reading).

Clearing the atmosphere

Offices and other work places can become very stuffy, with the air full of everybody else's smells – aftershave; hair-spray; coffee; egg sandwiches; cigarette smoke; photocopier chemicals; etc., and this can contribute to a lack of efficiency as the day wears on. Fresh air is what is needed, and if you cannot go out for a walk or fling open the windows, you can still freshen the atmosphere quite simply by sprinkling a few drops of an essential oil around you. Light citrousy oils like **rosewood**, **lemon**, **bergamot** or **melissa**; not only scent the atmosphere, but bring a freshness and clarity, and because all essential oils have antiseptic properties, will also offer you some measure of protection from the various airborne bacteria with which we are surrounded.

Anyone who is subject to 'off' days, when the slightest provocation can turn you into a 'weeping willow', can take comfort from **clary sage** oil. It is known as a euphoric oil and I know of people getting quite 'high' from smelling it. But when you are feeling low it just takes you back to a level of being in control of your emotions; and its prudent use has often helped me cope with emotional trauma.

Nervous diarrhoea

Have you ever had to keep rushing to the loo with an upset stomach, just before an important occasion. You know you haven't eaten anything terrible, so it must just be 'nerves'. But how can you stop it from happening? **Geranium** oil is sedative and uplifting at the same time, and is used by doctors in Italy to treat anxiety states. Two or three drops of the oil, on brown sugar or mixed into honey water (see page 120), and taken at hourly intervals for a couple of hours prior to the event, will soon bring relief whether you are going for an interview, starting a new job, or having your prospective 'in-laws' to dinner. **Neroli** oil, taken in the same way, will work just as effectively. It is preferable to add the essence to warm, sweetened water as the essential oils then reach the blood-stream very quickly, and bring very fast relief.

Muscular aches

Many more women now take part in physical activities, such as dancing, aerobic exercise, judo, squash, etc., than at any other time in the recent past. But have you ever over-done it a bit? When every muscle in your legs aches, and walking upstairs becomes an endurance test? It is at times like these, that I recommend a massage of the affected part (calf, thigh, shoulder, etc.) to bring relief, and speed up the repair process which goes on inside our muscles every time we strain them.

Of course, athletes and professional sports people always have a massage after their training sessions, but

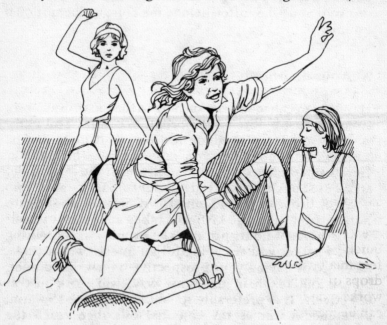

few of us are privileged to have our own personal physiotherapist, and so it becomes necessary and practical to take care of our own bodies and become our own 'physio'. Massage of the legs should always be in a circular movement, and always upwards towards the heart, never downwards to the feet. The pain experienced in the muscles is caused by a build-up of lactic acid, and by massaging the affected muscle, or groups of muscles, starting off gently and gradually applying more pressure, as the pain can be tolerated, the lactic acid is encouraged to disperse that much quicker. The massage alone will ease the pain and stiffness, and help to restore suppleness to the limbs, but for an even more effective treatment I would always recommend the addition of essential oils in a base oil, and you will find in the recipe section a blend which has been found to be of great help.

Aching feet

Our feet have a lot of weight to carry around, and often walk many miles in the course of a day. Naturally, if we all wore hiking boots and socks then our feet would not suffer in the same way that they do in high heels. But not many of us wish to hike around the supermarket or department store, and feet do get badly treated. When you realize that every part of your body has a reflex on the foot you begin to see that it is no wonder a pre-Christmas shopping trip can make us irritable, sick or headachy. Obviously there is no magic cure you can take whilst you are out, but on reaching home you can revive quite quickly by having a foot-bath. Just ten minutes with your feet in a bowl of water, to which you have first added six drops of **peppermint** oil, and gently massaging the feet, works wonders. Our feet have many reflex zones which can be massaged gently for a few minutes. Other oils that

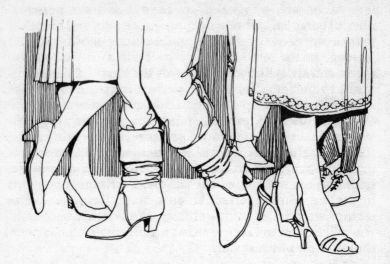

are just as effective are **lavender**, or **rosemary**. Again three to six drops will be needed.

Unwinding after a tiring day

Many things can 'wind us up'. Driving, coping with children, attending to countless customers in shops, commuting on a packed train, or doing whatever stressful occupation is pertinent to our lifestyle. The usual method of relaxation employed by people in the Western world has always been regular use of alcohol and cigarettes, but increasingly it is now tranquillizers. A more healthy and safe alternative to these measures is to take an aromatic bath each day. Even if you prefer showering for its speed and economy, think of bathing as a therapy and try to take one or two aromatic baths every week. Just as swimming in a warm sea is mentally and physically therapeutic, so too is lying in a warm aromatic bath, doing absolutely nothing except to inhale the vapours as they are released into the room. A few drops of your favourite essential oil (in particular **neroli; lemongrass; geranium;** or **lavender**) will soothe and gently ease away the mental and physical tensions of the day. It is, of course, as tension that the day's events register, and from there we get tight neck muscles, headaches, irritability and sometimes, insomnia. In Britain, thousands of women every week are prescribed tranquillizers, and although the prescription is supposed to be a short-term medication, the truth is that tranquillizers are addictive, and many women carry on taking these drugs for years. I find this very sad. I am sure that I have had my share of problems and mental anguish, and I know how well aromatherapy can help in overcoming life's setbacks. If we feel good within ourselves then the outside pressures never penetrate as deeply, or wound as hurtfully, as when we are feeling 'low' and vulnerable. For me, using essential oils is not only therapeutic on a physical level, but also on a mental and emotional one.

This is when the use of essential oils can and does justify its 'alternative to tranquillizers' claim. Although the use of, say **geranium** oil, in the bath or worn as a perfume, will reduce tension and harmonize troubled emotions, and **ylang-ylang** baths will lift depression, they are not harmful and will not produce any side-effects, and of course are non-addictive. In France, many doctors prescribe essential oils to their patients, alongside the usual array of drugs. Hopefully, that situation will become commonplace here in the not too distant future.

Insomnia

I no longer suffer from insomnia, but I have in the past, and

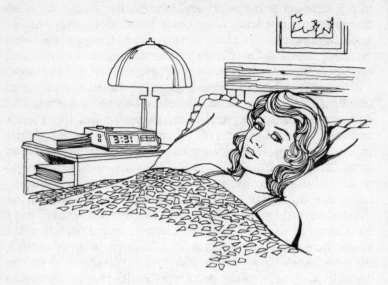

know just how frustrating it is to be in bed late at night and not be able to sleep. It is tension, both mental and physical, which causes us to stay 'switched on' instead of being able to naturally fall asleep. Some essential oils have sedative properties, and these can aid us in our efforts to switch off at night. For anyone suffering from insomnia it is advisable to take a leisurely bath, about an hour before bedtime, to which you have added four or five drops of **lavender** oil. Don't wash and scrub – this bath is not for cleanliness, it is for rest and relaxation; so just lie back and wallow, and don't set a time limit on yourself, stay as long as you feel comfortable, adding more hot water as necessary. After leaving the bath, put one drop of **neroli** oil on the edge of your pillow, or on to a tissue, and place it where you can smell it. Then just go to bed, and breathe in the vapours.

A friend of mine, who has been an insomniac for many

years, finds that oil of lavender helps her to sleep better than anything she has previously tried. If she happens to wake up in the night, she puts a drop of **lavender oil** on a tissue, pulls the sheet over her head, and soon drops off again.

Common sense must play a part in treating insomnia, and eating the main meal of the day at lunchtime, instead of in the evening, may help considerably. Also, some foods are best avoided, such as coffee, chocolate, and any stimulants which could hinder the daily 'slowing down' process of the body.

An even more powerful sedative oil is **marjoram**, although the smell is not so pleasant as lavender or neroli. A bath with three or four drops of marjoram oil or a drop on the edge of the pillow, will invariably ensure a good night's sleep.

Waking up in the night

Sometimes the day's events, or a particular worry, are so strongly entrenched in our minds that even when asleep, the slightest provocation (a cat fight in the garden, or a passing car) can awaken us, and it seems impossible to go back to sleep again. This happened to me quite recently. That day, I had been talking over a new business project, without having reached a satisfactory conclusion. I was awoken by my daughter visiting the loo, and thereafter lay in bed with half-baked plans constantly going through my mind. After half an hour or so, I realized that I was wasting time, and decided to put my thoughts down on paper. As soon as I had done this, and there was no danger of forgetting anything by the morning, I reached for my bottle of **lavender** oil, put a few drops on a tissue, and soon dropped off to sleep. (**Linden blossom, neroli,** or **marjoram** would have been just as effective.) Because there is such a temptation to want to stay warm and inert, I keep a notebook and pencil within reach of my pillow, just in case.

Revitalize before a night out

Sometimes your battery feels really flat and you are in sore need of an evening doing nothing to fully recharge, but the diary reminds you that you have a date, or a party to attend. Run a bath, and add either **rosemary** and **rosewood**, or **rosemary** and **bergamot**, or **rosewood** and **bergamot**; or just a single essence will suffice. Any of these essences or combinations will uplift and energize, and none of the aromas will interfere with your favourite perfume as they will evaporate from your skin soon after leaving the bath. If your body is now feeling revitalized and ready to go, but your head is still not enthusiastic, take two or three drops of **clary sage** oil in honey water. It works better than a glass of champagne, and has the added advantage of not causing your cheeks to flush!

Hangover

Most adults have, at some time or another, experienced a hangover. That unique combination of heavy head, thumping pain, nausea, foul taste in the mouth, photophobia (dislike of light), and generally feeling like death. This is hardly surprising, when you consider that alcohol is actually a poison when taken in excess, disturbing the body chemistry and robbing it of vital fluids. Run a warm bath, and in the meantime take a dose of **rose** and **peppermint** oil (one drop of each on brown sugar, or preferably in warm honey water), or alternatively take two drops of **fennel** oil. Then have a long drink of water and relax in the aromatic bath (see recipe section). If you do not have access to a bath, then you should massage a little **lavender** oil into the nape of the neck, and lie down with a **geranium** compress across the forehead.

2.
GYNAECOLOGICAL REMEDIES

Period pains

Menstruation is not an ailment to be cured, as women are destined to bleed every month for a large part of their lives. However, the accompanying pain and discomfort can be alleviated.

Maybe the pain is only discernible on the first day of a period, or perhaps the discomfort is so great that you have to go to bed for a day or two. Over the years I have taken the recommended homoeopathic remedies, but the thing which works for me, month after month, is **clary sage** oil. I take three drops in honey water at the onset of my period, when the pain is at its worst. Sometimes I need a second dose a few hours later, sometimes one dose is all that is required, but I am always amazed at how quickly the pain disappears and the heavy 'depressing' feeling is also lifted. Occasionally I 'test' the power of **clary sage**, by *not* taking it one month. The pain, irritability and depressed feelings which I then experience are tangible evidence that I do gain relief only with the use of **clary sage**. If an oral dose of **clary sage** is not wanted, then blend some **clary** with vegetable oil and massage the lower abdomen, inner thighs and lower back instead.

Premenstrual tension

Many women become tense and irritable a few days prior to the monthly 'curse'. Some women become unbearable to live with, and I have read of cases where murder has been committed at this particular time of month. Another manifestation of PMT or PMS (premenstrual syndrome) is a greater susceptibility to becoming upset and tearful. **Ylang-ylang** baths with an added drop of **lavender** or **clary sage**, each evening for the duration of the premenstrual symptoms, is sufficiently uplifting and soothing to make life a little more bearable all round. I do get 'weepy' and, although there is nothing wrong with a little cry, the embarrassing thing for me is not being able to stop. This is when I plunge into a **lemongrass** bath and wallow in the tangy vapours until I feel strengthened (usually twenty to thirty minutes.) If this is not practical, then a few drops of **clary sage** oil on a tissue helps me to gain control.

Water retention

Our body's ability to eliminate waste liquids is largely determined by the healthy functioning of our kidneys. On those days of the month when water retention becomes apparent – when you can't get your jeans done up, or your skirt button has to be unfastened – a diuretic can be employed to help you feel comfortable again. Many foods (vegetables in particular) have diuretic properties, but I like to take a bath in **juniper** oil, or take a drop of **juniper** in honey water, as I find this to be convenient and fast acting – and I am able to wear my favourite jeans at any time of the month.

Cystitis

This annoying and distressing problem is caused by an infection in the bladder or kidneys. Urinating is an unpleasant, often painful, experience and the burning sensation when passing water is often accompanied by pain further up inside the abdomen. **Juniper** or **camomile** may be taken in honey water (one drop of *either* of the essences). **Sandalwood** oil may also be rubbed in the kidney region of the lower back. If the discomfort is very bad, then I recommend a sitz bath with **lavender** oil, after each visit to the toilet, if this is practical. If you have still to go to work, then you could make up a bottle of **lavender** water each day to take with you (see page 108). A cotton wool pad impregnated with **lavender** water applied after going to the toilet, will give temporary local relief and help you to maintain your sanity. All strong food and drink should be avoided (tea, coffee, alcohol, spices, etc.) and a healthy diet, consisting of salads and grains, should be followed. I once suffered dreadfully from cystitis but, since becoming a vegetarian and a regular user of essential oils, I have not had a single attack.

Thrush (*candida albicans*)

This common complaint is extremely irritating to the mucous membranes of the outer vagina, and can seem almost to drive you insane. In my early twenties I suffered recurrent bouts of thrush, and each time I visited my doctor I was given a medicated pessary which brought temporary relief. However, I was never cured and thought that perhaps I was destined to have thrush for the remainder of my life. It was not until later, after treating myself with essential oils, that I could say with all honesty that I was *cured*. My choices of essence were **rose, lavender** and **bergamot**. (See page 108). I bought an enema pot from a chemist, and to 1 litre (1¾ pints) of warm water I added the essences. This douching of the vagina was repeated twice a day, until the water coming back out was completely clear. This took about a week, but the relief from itching was noticeable even from the first treatment. Thereafter I douched myself once a week for a further month. Douching should not be routinely employed as it will destroy the natural acid balance inside the vagina but, when used for periodic treatment of a particular complaint, it is very beneficial.

Herpes

Herpes, being a virus, cannot be 'knocked out' with anti-biotics, and the condition can be made better or worse by the general state of health of the sufferer. Several essential oils are of use in the treatment of genital herpes. **Lavender** baths, taken regularly, will stimulate the body's immune system, thereby aiding your body to fight the virus. **Eucalyptus** sitz baths will help, too, and a friend of mine was also given a **rose** blend to rub into the glands at the tops of the legs, and reported a marked improvement in her energy levels, and the lessening of the pain she had been experiencing. (See page 107.)

Pruritus

Pruritus means itching, and can pertain to the anus or the vagina. The saying 'there's no smoke without fire' could be translated as 'where there's an itch there's a problem'.

The problem could be purely an external irritant factor and it is never advisable to spray perfume or toilet waters near the vagina. Nor should one enter a bath to which essential oils have been added, without first ensuring that they are dispersed by agitating the water.

If the itching is caused by an infection, then see the relevant subheadings of this chapter, and treat it accordingly. Sometimes the fault can be traced back to an item of food which has been eaten, or to drinking excess quantities of alcohol. If, however, the itch is not accompanied by a discharge, and the mucous membranes are dry, try a daily lavender and rose sitz bath. (See page 108).

Leucorrhoea

A light vaginal discharge is quite normal. But prolonged, excessive discharge indicates that something is wrong with the general health of the body.

The vaginal discharge may be an indication of a food allergy. I am allergic to dairy products, and if I succumb to temptations when eating out, the immediate repercussion is a discharge. So I monitor my diet, and avoid those foods which cause problems.

Our bodies will tell us a lot, if we can only observe the signs, and act accordingly. If the discharge is troublesome, then it may be treated as described under the heading Pruritus or with a **lavender, bergamot** and **rose** douche.

Note: Many problems of the vagina could be due to the spine being in need of slight adjustment, and if you are troubled with lower back pain I recommend that treatment be sought from a McTimony chiropractor (see page 125).

3.
SEXUALITY AND SENSUALITY

Aphrodisiacs

A prerequisite to sexual expression is healthy sexual organs. How can you hope to feel sexy, if you are suffering from thrush, leucorrhea, herpes, or any one of the other

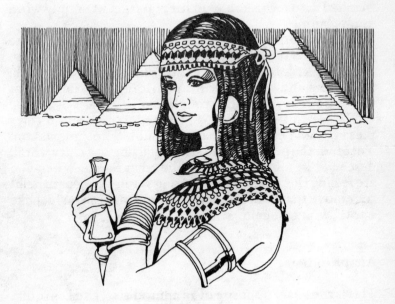

vaginal problems. The first thing is to get your body back to a state of health (see Chapter 2), and maintain that healthy state with correct diet.

The next important factor is being 'in the right mood' and it is here that essential oils can play a useful and welcome part. Our sense of smell is vital to our awareness, and it is this sense which has the closest link to our emotions. We can be 'put off' by 'turned on' by what we smell, even more so than by what we see. After all, it is easy to close one's eyes and let imagination take over, but we cannot close off our sense of smell. Many essential oils do not fit into the category of 'aphrodisiac' – namely the medicinal smelling ones, like eucalyptus – but there are many essences which excite the senses and register in the brain as being a 'turn on', and these include **ylang-ylang, jasmine, sandalwood, patchouli, rose,** and **clary sage**. These essences can be added to the bath water, sprinkled around a room, blended into a vegetable oil for massage, or simply worn as a perfume.

A massage between lovers is highly enjoyable. Some essential oils do serve to put you in the mood, and these essences, combined with gentle massage of the back, legs, arms and hands, etc., is physically relaxing and, at the same time, sexually stimulating.

We are all sensual beings, created to give and receive pleasure, and each of us has an inbuilt 'flame' of passion. Yet often the pressures and strain of living in a crazy world, descend like a blanket to smother that flame. When you are feeling this way, a long lingering **ylang-ylang** bath helps to remove that blanketed feeling, and makes you feel like a total woman again.

Anaphrodisiac

This is the exact opposite of an aphrodisiac, and I am quite sure that anyone who did not believe in aphrodisiacs would also not believe that an essential oil could 'turn them off'. However, **marjoram** oil – as well as being a strong sedative – has the power to turn off sexual desire.

Party atmosphere

To create a light, euphoric atmosphere in preparation for a party, sprinkle **clary sage** around the room, or put a few drops into a bowl of warm water. Having lived and worked with essential oils for many years, I take them completely for granted, but visitors always comment on the aromas, and you can live with the scents of freshly picked flowers and herbs, rather than the normal range of household smells.

Essential oils can be chosen according to the 'mood' of the party or the occasion. Here are some suggestions:

bergamot and **rosewood** for an impromptu summer's
  night party or disco
frankincense for a Christmas party
ylang-ylang for a St Valentine's Day party
sandalwood (or patchouli) to create an exotic oriental
  atmosphere for a special meal
orange for a children's party
geranium (or **rosewood**) for an afternoon tea
rose for a teenage girl's party

The permutations are endless and only subject to our personal preferences.

Confidence booster

A 'stiff drink' is the good old standby for nervousness about going somewhere new, or meeting someone for the first time, but what does a non-drinker do?

Jasmine has the power to inspire strength and confidence in the wearer, and is one of the most exquisite and precious essential oils. In the time of the pharaohs of Ancient Egypt, only the privileged few would be able to wear such a fragrance, and even today **jasmine** is 'rare' in comparison to say, **orange** or **lemon** oil. It is still expensive to purchase but, because of its heady fragrance and long lasting quality, it makes for a good 'investment'.

Perfume your lingerie

To give your lingerie your own 'personality', try adding one drop of your favourite essence to the rinsing water, the next time you hand-wash. Or sprinkle essential oils on to a cotton wool ball, put it inside a greaseproof bag, and place this in a drawer. A variation on the traditional lavender bag would be to make cotton bags and place a

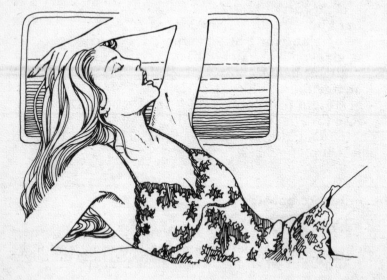

tissue or some cotton wool inside, which has first been impregnated with your favourite essential oil. Use long lasting scents such as **ylang-ylang, patchouli, geranium, linden blossom** or **rose**, rather than light, citrousy scents which are more 'volatile'. In Victorian times, when cashmere shawls were imported from Kashmir in India, they were packed in boxes containing **patchouli** leaves, as the smell discouraged moths. The same is true today, and many essential oils will protect clothing from the ravages of moths.

Note: Never apply essential oils directly onto clothing as permanent stains could result.

Breast enlarger

Evidence has been put forward to suggest that some plants contain 'phyto-hormones' (plant hormones) and that these work in a similar way to human hormones, which are responsible for many functions, including the development of the breasts. **Geranium** is purported to be very rich in these phyto-hormones and so, after a friend of mine had stopped breast-feeding her last child and found that she had reverted to a pre-pubescent bust measurement, I decided to put the theory to the test and gave her a blend of **geranium** and **ylang-ylang** in vegetable oil. The mixture (see page 108) was rubbed in, night and morning and, although still nowhere near to a 'playgirl of the month' appearance, she is pleased that the theory is proving to be true!

Thigh slimmer

Diet alone will never remove unwanted fat from the thighs,

and exercise is very important, perhaps even more so than counting calories. Certain essential oils, however, when massaged in, will aid the elimination of excess water from the thighs and buttocks. Regular use of an essential oil blend, including **juniper** which is a diuretic, will tone up the circulation, and de-toxify the body, thereby aiding your body's chemistry and capability of removing superfluous fat deposits. Bodily sluggishness will result in a sluggish circulation and poor lymphatic drainage, and revitalization of the person becomes necessary before slimming can hope to be successful. Therefore, a sensible attitude to exercise and diet will be necessary for successful slimming.

A slimming oil (see page 108) should be gently rubbed into the chosen areas every evening for a week or so, and always in an upward movement (towards the heart). The flesh should never be pummeled or pinched if cellulite is suspected, as violent treatment will only make the condition worse. Cellulite is the 'orange peel' appearance of the skin found on the thighs. The massage oil should be stroked from the knees to the hips in firm but gentle movements.

Making your own perfume

Our sense of smell is the most direct way in which our emotions can be triggered. It is also, in many people, the most neglected sense, and is often abused. Olfaction (to give it its technical term) registers in our brain, and we react with pleasure or displeasure according to what we have smelled.

We are all surrounded by unpleasant smells such as car exhaust fumes, and we like to compensate by donning more pleasing smells, such as deodorants, hair sprays, colognes and perfumes.

At one time, every perfume would have been skilfully blended from the finest essential oils, and would indeed have been a delight and an indulgence (on the pysche, and on the purse). Sadly, with the advent of laboratory produced 'floral' chemicals, perfumes have become more and more synthetic. Very expensive perfumes still use larger amounts of essential oils, having been created out of years of practice in the art of perfumery. You can make quite passable perfumes yourself, by blending together a few drops of your favourite essences. You obviously will not be able to create a sophisticated perfume, but you will find that simple perfumes can be concocted, and worn with pride (see pages 109 and 110).

Alcohol is the usual medium in which a perfume is diluted, but pure alcohol is not for sale to the general public. Vodka or gin could be used if you don't mind smelling like a cocktail. Vegetable oils, because of their oxidizing qualities, (that is they 'go off') are not suitable. However, *jojoba* oil, being a *liquid wax*, and not being subject to oxidation, is the ideal base in which to dilute your perfumes. It is a little greasy, and you will just need to rub a small amount behind the ears, knees, on wrists or wherever you choose.

For hot summer days, you could make your own '*cologne*' for splashing on liberally. It is quite simple to make by blending together a number of essential oils (see page 110), adding them to water (bottled or distilled) and shaking vigorously. This is delightfully cooling and refreshing, and inexpensive.

Turn your bedroom into a 'boudoir'

With lashings of essential oils and a little imagination you could be Cleopatra, Madame Pompadour, or whoever you want to be. Essential oils were the only perfumes available

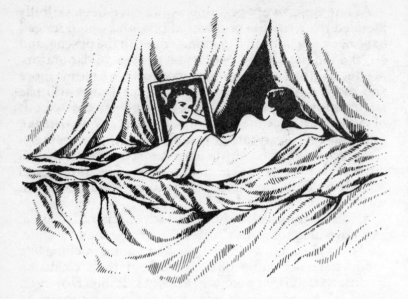

in times gone by, because synthetic aromas had not been invented. The ancient Egyptian barges were often drenched in aromatic oils and fragrant waters and, in Roman palaces, rose water was poured into the canals running through the gardens. Cleopatra was reputed to have seduced Mark Antony by wearing **jasmine** oil at their business meetings. Certain essential oils have 'heady' euphoric qualities, so why not take your favourites and sprinkle them liberally around the bedroom!

The heavier perfume notes of these oils could seem to be more suited to bedrooms and seduction because their odour is close to that of natural body scent, whereas the light citrousy oils are reminiscent of the fresh outdoors and open spaces.

Rose must surely be the favourite perfume of all time. It has been used throughout the centuries, and still is today in practically every high class perfume. **Rose otto** has always been costly, and will always be so, due to the very small yield of essential oil from each flower. However, although the cost is high in comparison to that of other essential oils, it is not prohibitively so, and it does have fantastic 'keeping' qualities. To my mind, **rose** is in a class of its own and no other scent makes me feel so special.

Other 'heady' essential oils are **ylang-ylang, patchouli, sandalwood, jasmine** and **linden blossom.**

4.
HEALTH AND HEALING

We cannot expect to look radiant and be brimming with health, if our stomachs are given 'rubbish' food with which to work. The face mirrors the health of the body in general, and the condition of our skin is not merely determined by what we put *on* it, or how thoroughly we cleanse it, but what we put *in* it: what we eat, what we drink, and our state of mind.

It is absolutely vital that our diet contains sufficient fibre. It is impossible to have a flawless complexion and be constipated at the same time. The skin is an organ, and is subject to ill health just as any other of our organs can suffer. Too much coffee will cause backache as the kidneys complain, and this is reflected in the face by dark circles and puffiness under the eyes. Too many dairy products in the diet can cause excess catarrh and sinus problems, amongst other things. A diet high in fried foods will usually be reflected by a greasy, spotty complexion. Too much alcohol will not only damage the liver eventually, but causes broken veins in the face.

Food allergies are now recognized as being responsible for much ill health, and recurrent bouts of trivial but

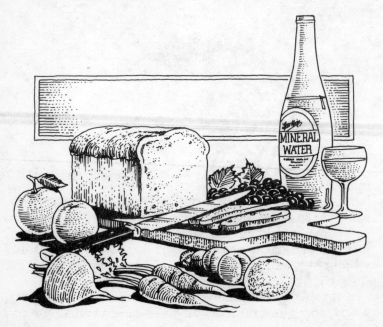

irritating symptoms. An allergy to a particular food is obviously a very individual thing; for example, although I have found that dairy products are responsible for a lot of the complaints I just accepted for years, I cannot assume that dairy products are bad for everyone.

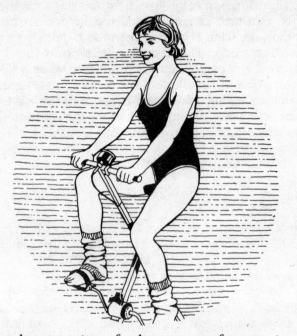

Regular exercise of whatever preference is of immeasurable benefit to our bodies. It stimulates the circulation of blood, which carries oxygen around our body, tones the muscles, massages the internal organs, and helps to keep the lymphatic system in a healthy condition. I know a man in his sixties who is incredibly healthy and vibrant by taking daily exercise, avoiding alcohol and sugary foods and only eating when he feels hungry.

A troubled mind is also revealed in the face. Fear, grief, worry, anger, resentment and depression all affect the way

we look. The expression 'green with envy' is supposed to
have come into use because of evidence that jealousy and
envy affect the liver, which regulates the flow of bile. And
every ailment from arthritis to cancer is now thought to
be affected by negative or positive states of mind. It makes
sense, therefore, to take fast, positive steps whenever a
negative emotion comes along, and I know of nothing
better than the Bach Flower Remedies for quickly restoring
positive emotions. There seems little point in allowing
disease to develop even to the point when it can be looked
at by a doctor and 'labelled'. If the problems are dealt with
promptly, then they may never advance to the stage when
they can be 'named'. Bach flower remedies, homoeopathy
and aromatherapy all help prevent the likelihood of serious
health problems.

Massage

Cats love to be stroked, dogs to be patted, children to be
cuddled – the sense of touch is important to us, and needs
satisfying.

We are all sensual beings and our bodies appreciate and
'warm' to a massage. Unfortunately, in this country,
massage has become almost a dirty word, and anyone calling
themselves a 'masseuse' is regarded with suspicion. But
some countries, notably Japan, regard massage as a part
of daily life. The 'geisha girls' are employed to serve the
needs of businessmen, not in a sexual way, but by serving
them food, playing music, and offering a massage. It is an
important part of the Japanese 'humility', to serve another
person.

The art of massage is essentially that of giving of oneself
to another person, and although the masseuse is obviously
expending more energy than the recipient, the giving of a
massage is as much a beautiful experience as is the receiving.

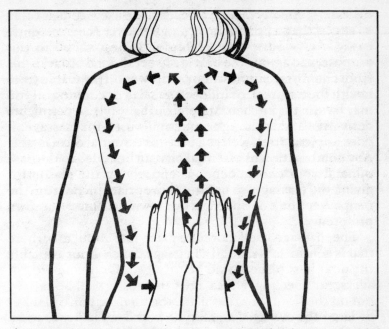

A massage incorporating some essential oils in a simple blend will enhance the treatment. A massage with a 'relaxing' blend of oils can bring about deep relaxation in an otherwise anxious person, and will ease and soothe away many of life's tensions. A massage with an 'invigorating' blend can enliven a depressed person, and bring back energy to someone who is exhausted and care-worn.

Practitioners of alternative medicine, including those specializing in massage, are becoming very popular now and, as it is not possible for a therapist to treat people without giving a lot of their time, patience and care, it would seem highly desirable for anyone suffering from depression or other chronic problem to consider seeking help from an aromatherapist. But it is also relatively easy to give someone a massage at home. It helps to have had a training in basic massage techniques, but it is not absolutely necessary. An oily medium needs to be used, so that there is 'slip' – that is, the hands can glide over the back quite easily. An odourless vegetable oil is best suited to this purpose, and among the best are sweet almond oil (available from chemists), sunflower or safflower oil (available from health food stores), or indeed any salad or cooking oil you may have in the kitchen. Mineral oil (baby oil) is a petroleum derivative and, although sometimes used for massage, it does not lend itself well as a base for essential oil massage. Any combination of essential oils can be added to the base oil, and your choice depends entirely on the reason for giving the massage, so use the appropriate blend from the recipe section, or invent your own to suit your own preferences.

The massage itself can take place just about anywhere that is comfortable, but if a massage couch is not available the next best place would be on a bed. Or, if you are not averse to kneeling, a massage can equally well be carried out on the floor, but first place the recipient on a blanket or large towel with a small pillow under the head, and a regular size pillow under the stomach if the recipient is of slim build. A plump person would probably not need the tummy pillow. Pregnant women, in their last few months, would find lying on their stomachs uncomfortable, and will find that lying on their side will enable the masseuse to rub their back quite effectively.

Everyone's skin is warm but a massage oil straight from a bottle is cold, so never pour the oil directly onto someone's back, as it will shock the system. It is best to pour some into the palm of the hand, and then rub your hands together before beginning the massage. Run your hands over the surface of the back to deposit oil evenly over the skin. Then, starting at hip level, place your hands on the back, palms down flat and fingers pointing up towards the head, and slide them smoothly but firmly up the spine until your fingers reach the nape of the neck. Then glide your hands sideways across the shoulders, and draw down towards where you started. This should be carried out as one continuous movement, for up to ten minutes, or less if you feel tired. At the end of the massage, cover the back area with a paper napkin or piece of kitchen roll, and press down lightly. This will remove any excess oil which has not been absorbed by the skin.

Note: Do not massage anyone who has cancer; an acute infection; a fever; a serious heart complaint, or has just eaten a big meal. Do not massage over varicose veins. It is not advisable to massage the genitals with an essential oil blend as it is an extremely sensitive area and skin irritation may result.

Depression

Depression is something that can strike any one of us. Sometimes there is a reason for the depression. Sometimes it descends for no reason, like a black cloud blotting out the light. If you have an acute attack of depression, as is most common, then a bath in **ylang-ylang** or **clary sage**, will go a long way towards making you feel better. **Jasmine** oil, although rather costly to buy, is a really excellent depression-fighter. It lifts the spirits, and makes you feel good. When depression becomes chronic then, as well as taking aromatic baths, it could be extremely helpful to visit a qualified aromatherapist. Someone who can sympathize, listen to you, and treat you with essential oils, tailored to your individual needs.

So many women rush to the doctor when depressed and, although they probably went along to the surgery hoping for a bit of comfort and understanding, unfortunately they very often leave with a prescription for anti-depressants. Doctors are usually overworked, and on top of that they may not be feeling too good themselves after talking to, and coping with, many people and their problems. It is worth the small investment, to see an aromatherapist, because when you are really depressed the effort of self-help may be beyond your reach.

Slimming

Essential oils can act as wonderful aids to the serious slimmer, if diet and exercise are also attended to. Often a sluggish circulation and/or water retention are problems which a fat person takes for granted, as well as a slow metabolic rate.

As **juniper** oil is a natural diuretic, it is helpful to have a **juniper** bath at least once a week. Used regularly it really does work by causing an increase in the flow of water from the body, and along with the liquid goes the toxic waste that, unless eliminated, builds up in the body of the over-weight person. For anyone with a small bust, but large hips and thighs, then it would be preferable to have a **juniper** hip bath – just sit in the bath, but don't lie down because you do not want to lose any weight from the breasts.

Fat people tend to overeat when feeling depressed about size or shape and, when an eating binge threatens, it would be preferable to have a **clary sage** and **ylang-ylang** bath. The uplifting aromatic waters may just give you enough of a lift to make you proud of yourself, and not want to take two steps back by eating excessive quantities of food.

Regular bathing with essential oils will improve the tone of the entire body, the clarity of the skin, and generally make you feel fitter and more determined to 'fight the flab'.

Take your healthy atmosphere with you

Hotel rooms seem to me to be the ideal place to catch a

variety of germs depending on what was wrong with the previous occupant. Whenever I need to stay in a hotel, I always take with me a selection of essential oils. Not only do the familiar smells make me feel 'at home', but I know that certain essential oils will safeguard my health, by killing the airborne bacteria. My personal preferences are **rosewood, bergamot,** and **lavender**. As soon as I arrive, I sprinkle one or more essences in the bathroom and on the carpet.

Mouth ulcers

Mouth ulcers generally occur when one is run down, and can also be attributed to excessive sugar consumption. It is wise to avoid sugary foods for a while, and treat the ulcer to a swab of **myrrh**. Put a drop of **myrrh** oil on the end of a cotton bud and apply gently to the ulcer. There is an initial sting, but very soon there is a complete relief of discomfort and the raw area is quickly healed. With this treatment several times a day, the mouth ulcers should not last more than a day or two at most.

Spots

Facial spots are caused either by clogged pores, faulty nutrition, a hormone imbalance (such as occurs during puberty) or an allergic reaction to some item of food. Sometimes spots occur just before or at the start of menstruation. Cleansing the skin is important, as is eating fresh foods and avoiding processed, chemically-coloured and flavoured foods. An increase in the amount of mineral water drunk will also be beneficial.

In the case of an acute outbreak of spots, a cotton bud dipped in either **camphor, eucalyptus** or **lavender** oil,

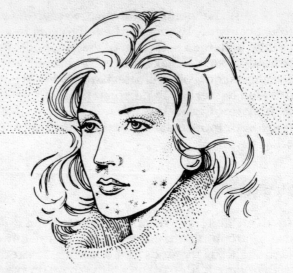

and applied directly to the spot, will often clear it up overnight. It is preferable to apply the oil at night so that the essence gets a chance to work without the presence of make-up.

Sunburn

The majority of us, at some time or other, have been unlucky enough to suffer the agonies of sunburn and, whilst slapping on the *après-sun* lotions, have vowed never again to underestimate the burning rays of the sun. If sunburn should occur, on reaching home or hotel add three drops of either **lavender** or **peppermint** oil to a tepid bath. This treatment will take out a lot of the heat, and soothe the burnt skin. **Lavender** can even be used neat on small areas of sunburn, such as the nose or shoulders, and a bottle of **lavender** is a 'must' for a holiday first-aid bag. If on holiday with only a shower available, a plant mist spray could be filled with lukewarm water plus a few drops of **lavender** oil. When this is sprayed over the sunburnt part of the body it brings immediate relief, and the spray can be repeated as soon as the relief wears off. It is also advisable to avoid drinking alcohol and instead to drink lots of mineral water or fruit juices, as the consumption of alcohol causes dehydration and you need to replace the moisture content which the sun has taken out.

Note: **Lavender** is the *only* essential oil I would apply neat to the skin.

Burns

Burns, whether caused by hot water or fire, can safely be treated in the same way as sunburn. A small burn will immediately feel better with a drop or two of **lavender** oil and this treatment can be repeated if the pain returns. A doctor should always be called to deal with larger burns but, whilst waiting for him, the affected part should be placed in a bowl of cold water to which ten drops of **lavender** has first been added.

Lavender diluted in vegetable oil, should never be used on a burn, as any fatty or oily substance will only cause the burn to feel hotter.

Lavender oil, either neat or in water, has the unique ability to reduce heat, minimize pain, aid rapid healing, and at the same time to calm the patient. Even a second degree burn has been known to heal within a week leaving no scarring when treated with this essential oil.

Foot baths

For relief from hot, swollen, aching feet, add five drops of

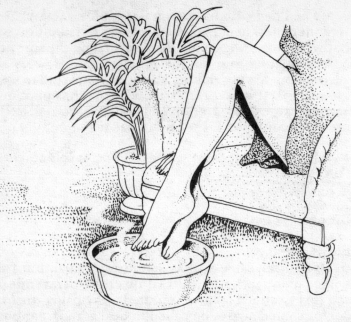

peppermint oil to a bowl of lukewarm water (or sit on the edge of the bath with a few inches of water in the bottom) and let the feet soak for fifteen minutes. **Peppermint** contains natural menthol which is incredibly cooling.

Smelly feet are an embarrassment to their owners, and this condition seems to affect men more than women, probably due to their feet being encased in thick socks and heavy shoes more frequently. **Cypress** oil is a natural deodorant, and when used regularly, minimizes the awful smell. Use six drops of the essential oil in a bowl of warm water.

Athlete's foot is a condition which occurs between the toes, caused by a fungus multiplying in a warm, moist place. I have found that a drop or two of **lavender** oil, massaged into the affected part of the foot, clears up a case of athlete's foot in a matter of days.

My son recently complained of pain in the ball of his foot, and it seemed that the latest visit to the swimming baths had resulted in a verruca. **Lavender** oil on a cotton bud was applied to the site, and this treatment was repeated several times during the day. This cleared up the condition very quickly, but equally effective would be **eucalyptus, rosemary** or **camphor** oil.

Fainting

When someone loses consciousness through fright, shock or exhaustion, something is required to jog the faint person back into consciousness, and any of the powerfully smelling essential oils, such as **rosemary, peppermint** or **basil** will perform this function. Recently, I read a newspaper article about **peppermint** oil being used to bring a boy out of a coma. This oil was placed on a piece of lint and wafted under the patient's nose – it worked!

Headache

Headaches are such a common occurrence that they are big business for the drug companies, who are always claiming a new fast-acting remedy. Sometimes a headache is caused by neck tension, and this can be relieved by massaging a little **lavender** oil into the muscles at the back of the neck. Often a spot of **lavender** oil gently rubbed in over the temples will bring relief from forehead pain associated with eye strain.

When a 'sick headache' strikes, then the best remedy is a dose of **peppermint** oil on sugar, or in honey water. Even **peppermint** oil, dripped on to a tissue and sniffed frequently, will dispel a headache caused by overeating or indigestion. Sometimes the best cure for a headache is just to go to bed and have a good sleep. This can be aided with a drop of **Lavender** or **neroli** on the pillow.

Indigestion and flatulence

For very fast acting relief to the discomforts of indigestion, take two or three drops of **peppermint** oil on sugar, or in honey water.

Flatulence can be treated very effectively with **fennel** oil. Just one or two drops on sugar or in honey water brings very fast relief.

Toothache

The age old remedy of **clove** oil being used for toothache holds just as good today. A drop of this oil on cotton wool, applied to the aching tooth, takes away much of the discomfort. **Clove** oil has a slight analgesic effect, and numbs the nerves in the local area of application. **Peppermint** oil is also a good remedy for toothache when applied to the affected tooth.

Haemorrhoids (piles)

Haemorrhoids are very painful and can strike anyone at some time or another. The chances of piles occuring are much greater if one is also suffering from constipation. **Cypress** oil (five drops in a bowl of warm water, or in the bath) will relieve the discomfort of haemorrhoids. In fact, many people have told me that their piles had simply shrunk and disappeared after a **cypress** bath. Please do not be tempted to apply **cypress** oil neat, as it is very strong and will only cause further discomfort. Always add the drops to water, and mix well before entering the sitz bath.

High blood-pressure (hypertension)

As **lavender** oil is sedative and has been attributed with the ability of lowering blood-pressure, I have recommended it to quite a few people suffering from high blood-pressure. My mother, who suffers from hypertension, takes regular **lavender** baths, especially when something has occurred to upset her and she feels 'hot and bothered'. **Lavender** baths always leave her feeling relaxed and calmed. Other essential oils which would be good to use are **marjoram** and **ylang-ylang**.

Influenza

I find that influenza responds very quickly to homoeopathic remedies but, when these are not readily available, there is an aromatic treatment which has the ability to abort a cold and shorten an influenza attack.

Fill a bath with comfortably warm water. Mix a quantity of **lavender** oil in a base oil (see page 120). Rub the mixture into your body, paying particular attention to the chest area and back of the neck. Then jump into the bath, and soak for about ten minutes. Dry quickly and go straight to bed.

This treatment will usually lessen the severity of attack, and in some cases it clears up the symptoms overnight.

Laryngitis/sore throat

Sandalwood oil has very powerful anti-bacterial properties and can kill streptococci and staphylococci as effectively as can antibiotics. Two or three drops in honey water, repeated every few hours, is a wonderful first-aid treatment for sore throats and laryngitis. **Sandalwood** oil also has a slight analgesic quality, and a very sore throat finds instant relief.

Note: It is vital that the **Sandalwood** oil is genuine Mysore, so only buy from a trusted company.

Colds and stuffiness

The symptoms of a cold are well known to everyone – sneezing, aching head, painful bones in the face, running or blocked nose, watery eyes, sore throat. Colds often spread to the chest as well, and the ill feeling is compounded by a sore chest, coughing and possibly even bronchitis.

Rather than allow the bacteria or virus to multiply and cause such misery, take some positive action at the onset of the cold. **Camphor** oil is fast acting and can often abort a cold in the early stages. One or two drops of **camphor** on brown sugar, repeated every two hours for three or four doses, should be sufficient. **Eucalyptus** oil on a tissue and sniffed regularly, or a few drops placed on the edge of a pillow, will often dry up a cold overnight.

Bathing regularly with essential oil of **lavender** will serve to build up resistance to colds and other infections, by increasing the body's production of healthy blood cells, and when **lavender** oil is used in the treatment of infection (in a bath or as a rub) it has the ability to stimulate the white blood cells, so that the invading organisms are destroyed faster.

Shingles

An adult whose health is below par can catch the chicken pox virus from a child. The manifestation may not be that of chicken pox, but of shingles. Here, a homoeopathic remedy should be sought, and the affected area bathed with **peppermint** lotion, as for chicken pox (page 117) or with dilute **geranium**.

Mouth wash

Bad breath is something that can occur from a variety of causes. Perhaps we have eaten spicy or strong-tasting food. Or were too busy to eat and just drank coffee instead. Persistent worry; illness; nervousness before an event – all these things and more can make us self-conscious about our breath. There are lots of mouth washes and mouth sprays available but they all have one thing in common, they are not natural. A mouth wash can be made in the same way as a floral water for the skin, except that the mouth wash can be stronger. Quite a few oils may be used, either singly or in combinations of two or three, these are **peppermint, basil, fennel, lemon, lavender, clary sage, bergamot, rose** and **ylang-ylang** (see page 111).

5.

SKIN AND HAIR CARE

Your face may not be your fortune, but a glowing, healthy skin is the basis for looking beautiful. Many women hide under their make-up, and won't be seen without it. But it really gives you confidence to know that, even when the skilfully applied make-up comes off at night, you still have a beautiful complexion and a good colour, free from spots and blemishes and soft to the touch. It does not take a lot of time or great deal of money to look good, just daily attention to nurturing and protecting the skin. Nature's repair process is slow and steady, with cells being constantly replaced. With the passing of the years this repair process slows down but, with the regular application of essential oils, this slowing down will not begin as soon. Because women have more fat in their tissues than do men, women's bodies absorb and retain essential oils to a greater degree than the average male, and this could account for the wonderful results achieved in beauty salons and homes around the country.

Real beauty comes from within. It is not something we can buy in pots, massage in, or obtain from a beauty salon. But it is something that can be acquired, as a whole person improves their state of health, vitality and confidence. In conjunction with a good diet, the use of essential oils on skin brings gradual improvement in the texture and appearance of the complexion. We don't have to accept what we see in the mirror. If we don't like what we see we can change it. I don't mean by plastic surgery because I don't think that wrinkles or a large nose make any difference to a person's beauty. Beauty comes from within and everyone has the power to possess healthy shining hair, sparkling eyes, and a happy countenance. For me, meditation is vitally important for my well-being and happiness, and has made a big difference to my life. I see the body as being like a car, and the person as the mechanic of the car. We can either 'tune up' and look after the vehicle or leave it to get rusty, and fall apart! According to a survey carried out in America, the thing that men found most exciting and attractive about a woman was not her face, or legs, or bosom, but the way she felt about herself, which was reflected in the way she carried herself. For this you need the confidence that comes with knowing that you look and feel good, feel sensual, even if you don't happen to look like a model or film star. That is the sex appeal we all have. There is more to being beautiful than having a pretty face. Perhaps you have an idol, or admire someone beautiful, but you can never look *like* that person, any more than you could change your finger prints. Everyone is unique, and special in their own way, and it is from that basic understanding, that we are as wretched or as beautiful as we experience ourself to be, that we can begin to improve. Miracles do not happen overnight. If a car has been neglected for many years then it will take a lot of attention before it can even be driven, let alone raced. Better by far, to care for your body, which is a gift you only have for a certain number of years on this earth.

Using essential oils on the skin

Essential oils are safe to use on the skin, providing that the following points are remembered:

1. Ensure that you are using true essential oils, and not a synthetic blend of aromatic substances labelled as essential oil. To be sure, always buy your essential oils from a reputable company that you know you can trust.

2. Never use neat essential oils on the face (with the exception of dabbing spots). Apart from being too concentrated, a vegetable oil is needed to disperse the essential oils, and also to provide 'spreadability'.

3. Never use a mineral oil (such as baby oil) with essential oils, as mineral oil will not penetrate the skin, and will inhibit the action of the essential oils.

4. Dilute the essential oils in a carrier oil. Use either sweet almond, apricot kernel, sunflower, soya, peanut oil or whatever salad oil you have. Olive oil tends to have a strong smell of its own, but may be used. **Wheat germ** oil, when added to a blend (10 per cent) will help to preserve it, as this oil contains a good percentage of vitamin E which acts as a natural anti-oxidant. If a blend is to be used within two or three days, then it is not necessary to include the **wheat germ** oil, unless you just want to add to the nourishing powers of the mixture.

5. For daily facial massage, a blend consisting of 98 per cent vegetable oil to 2 per cent essential oil, is ideal. (See page 120).

6. If your hand should accidentally slip whilst adding drops of essential oil to the base oil, and more drops of essence are added than you intended, simply add more vegetable oil to compensate.

How essential oils work through the skin

The beauty of an aromatherapy facial, or facial massage

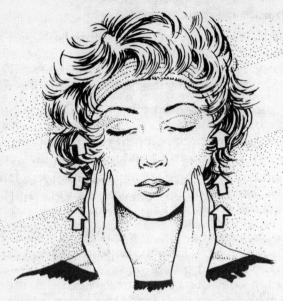

with an essential oil blend, is that it is not merely a 'topical' application, but a real treatment which works on a deeper level.

Essential oils, because of their volatile nature, have the ability to penetrate through the skin to the dermis, the underlying layers of the skin. Essential oils travel through the interstitial fluids, blood-stream and lymphatic system.

It is possible to effect a remarkable change in the condition of the skin by applying a treatment oil each night before going to bed. A gentle massage with light, upward movements, is all that is really necessary to acquire a flawless complexion and then to maintain it.

Treatment of acne and teenage problem skins

Spots and acne usually stem from puberty, when the

hormone changes in the body produce substances which, if not eliminated via the kidneys, liver and skin will build up and cause eruptions on the face and neck, and occasionally on other parts of the body too. I know that antibiotics are routinely prescribed for this condition, but it seems to me to be adding fuel to the fire. I am not a doctor, but I sense that the entire body needs to be detoxified, and feel that this can only be achieved with a combination of good diet, blood purifying herbal tablets, and essential oils massaged into the skin and added to the bath. The temptation to apply astringents or squeese spots should be avoided, as these methods will not cure the condition, and will only stimulate the sebaceous glands to work overtime, and also encourage the spread of bacteria.

A nightly facial massage with a blend for acne (see page 112) will work on a deep level, imparting a natural antiseptic to the infected areas, and at the same time regulating the secretion of sebum.

Many times I have been asked, 'But how can an *oil* get rid of *oily* skin'. It can because, as explained earlier, the vegetable oil is merely a spreading agent, and it is essential oils which are going to work on the problem. Essential oils are 'the hidden workers' and, whilst you sleep, a healing and normalizing action is taking place.

After thorough cleansing, a liberal amount of the 'acne blend' should be gently massaged into the face and neck, each night before going to bed. After ten minutes, place a tissue over the face and press gently. This will remove any excess oil that has not been absorbed by the skin. Very toxic skins will not absorb much oil but, if used regularly over a period of time, the skin's improvement will show itself with more of the oil being absorbed. Do not expect a flawless complexion within a fortnight, but treat your skin every night and you will soon begin to notice a difference in appearance and texture.

Dry skin

A hot climate, illness or bad diet can all affect the skin, causing it to feel and look dry and taut. Dry skin becomes wrinkled more easily than greasy skin, and needs daily nourishing. Moisturizing creams, although useful to apply before going out in the morning, are not really going to make much impact on a dry complexion. A special blend of essential oils, chosen for their ability to nourish and improve the skin (see page 112), should be gently massaged into the face and neck every night before going to bed. For people with very dry skin, the same mixture could be used in the morning under make-up. I like to apply the oil blend immediately after toning my skin with rosewater, whilst the skin is still moist. This is my 'moisturizer'.

Mature skin

As we grow older, our skin cells do not renew themselves quite as quickly as when we were children. However, because some essential oils have the capability of speeding up the re-growth of skin cells, we could rightly call them rejuvenators.

Essential oils which fall into this category are; **neroli, myrrh, rose, frankincense** and **lavender**. A massage blend should be made up (see page 112), and the face and neck massaged every night. The essential oils will work on the underlying tissues whilst you are sleeping and, if used regularly for a period of time, you will notice a vast improvement.

After gently massaging the oil into the face and neck, avoiding the eye area, a **neroli** compress (see page 113) may be applied over the face to aid penetration of the oils, whilst at the same time relaxing you.

Floral waters

It is very simple and cheap to make your own floral waters (see page 112). These waters are ideal to tone and freshen your face after cleansing, or any time during a hot summer's day. Alcohol is not good for the skin, and so it is better not to include it in the making of a floral water. Tap water is not suitable for making a floral water as it contains too many chemicals and other organisms. Always use a bottled spa water whenever possible.

It has become popular, of late, to spray the face with mineral water. I have an aversion to aerosol sprays, and prefer to make a floral water, and then add it to a clean, empty mist spray and lightly spray my face. Again, you will need to renew the aromatic water every two or three days, but it is a very simple task.

Facial masks

Every now and again it is beneficial to have a facial mask, which will draw impurities to the surface of the skin, and stimulate circulation. There are a great many available in the shops, but it is fun to make one's own (see page 113). If your skin is very greasy, then you may safely leave the mask until it dries. However, if you have dry skin the mask should be removed after ten minutes. To remove the mask, just soak cotton wool in warm water and wipe over the face. Continue using fresh cotton wool as necessary, until the face is clean again.

To counteract any possible drying effects of the mask, apply a little facial massage oil to the skin. Or alternatively, rub in a little **rose** body perfume.

Eye compresses

Tired eyes, or those irritated by contact lenses, or from being in a smoky atmosphere, will find immediate relief from a **camomile** or **lavender** compress. Put one drop of the essence into a bowl of cold water (large enough to hold 1 litre), mix well and after soaking two cotton wool pads, squeeze out excess liquid and place one on each eye. Lie down for ten minutes whilst the compress is soothing your eyes.

Body rubs

Keep your body looking great, and smelling divine, whilst giving it the protection of the therapeutic powers of **rose** (see page 113). Just rub a little into the skin after bathing or showering. Be a little more generous with neck, elbows, and any parts of the body which tend towards dryness and are looking aged.

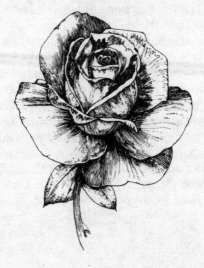

Jojoba oil

Jojoba oil, though not an absolutely vital ingredient, is a super emollient. It is not a vegetable oil but a liquid wax, and when incorporated into a massage oil for the face or body it imparts a satin-smooth quality to the skin. Up to now, whales have been hunted and killed for their oil (spermaceti) which is used in cosmetics for its emollient properties. Now there is no need to hunt a creature to extinction for the sake of beauty, as the jojoba nut provides the same emollience for the skin. Much research is being carried out regarding the benefits of jojoba, but American Indian tribes have for centuries been employing jojoba oil for skin complaints, on both dry and greasy skins, and as a protection and conditioner for their hair.

Hair rinses

The use of any essential oil in a hair rinse will impart a lovely natural smell to the hair, but some essential oils are particularly good for different hair colourings. Make up a jug of **rosemary** rinse (see page 114) and, after washing hair in the usual way, pour the rinse through the hair and then dry as normal. This will bring lustre and depth to dark hair.

For fair hair, a **camomile** rinse can be made in the same way (see page 114) and poured through the hair after washing as usual. This has a natural lightening effect on fair hair and, at the same time, will improve the condition of dry, bleached hair.

Oil treatment for damaged hair

Hair that has been damaged by weather, perming or

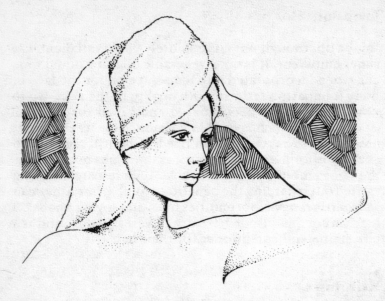

bleaching, can be improved by a once-a-week oil treatment. The hair should be parted in sections and the blend for damaged hair (see page 114) should be applied along the partings. Then, taking a piece of cotton wool which has been dipped in the oil, stroke down to the ends of the hair.

When all the hair has been saturated, pile the hair on top of the head and wrap in a towel. A minimum of two hours should elapse before washing off the oil, and shampoo should be applied to the hair and worked in before water is added. If water is added first, it becomes very difficult to remove all the oil.

Treatment for greasy hair

Make up the recipe on page 113, then proceed as for damaged hair (above).

Treatment for head lice

Make up the recipe on page 114 then proceed as for head lice, on page 102.

Dandruff treatment oil

Make up the recipe on page 114, then proceed as for damaged hair (page 72).

Conditioner for normal hair

To impart an incredible shine to normal hair, take some good quality vegetable oil, add jojoba oil and the essential oil of your choice. (See page 120). Massage through the hair, paying particular attention to the ends, especially on long hair, where split ends could be a problem. Pile the hair up and wrap in a towel. Leave on for thirty minutes to an hour and then wash off, adding shampoo before water. A once-weekly treatment, will condition hair beautifully, and add a lustre that ordinary conditioners don't quite manage.

6.
PREGNANCY AND CHILDBIRTH

Contra-indications

Certain oils should be avoided during pregnancy or if you think you may be pregnant; these are cinnamon bark, basil, pennyroyal, hyssop, myrrh, savoury, sage, thyme and origanum.

Nausea

There is nothing safer or more effective to take for morning sickness than **peppermint** oil; either on brown sugar, or in honey water. Nausea is a very common problem in the early stages of pregnancy, but it is easily remedied with a sensible diet, and peppermint oil (or even peppermint tea, several times a day if you prefer). There is no necessity to seek relief with prescribed drugs, and the thalidomide tragedies would never have occurred, if doctors and ante-natal classes had recommended their pregnant patients to take herb teas and essential oils, instead of inconclusively tested chemicals.

A drop of peppermint, taken every hour until relief is obtained (maybe a single dose per day will be sufficient) is usually adequate to bring relief, but in very severe cases where the woman constantly vomits, then it would be preferable to take a homoeopathic remedy (such as

Ipecacuanha) and apply a **lavender** compress to the abdomen. This is quite simple to do. Add two drops of lavender to a bowl of warm water. Soak a small towel and wring it out, then apply to the abdomen. Place a larger dry towel over the top, and rest for thirty minutes or so.

Pregnant women are very sensitive to smells, and during my pregnancies I liked to surround myself with a healthy, scented atmosphere. My favourite essences were **bergamot, geranium , lavender, rose,** and **linden blossom.** I would pour a few drops of one of them into a bowl of hot water and let the vapours fill the atmosphere. All essential oils have anti-bacterial properties, and they do afford a considerable degree of protection from undesirable airborne bacteria. One day, in the not too distant future, I hope to see aromatherapeutic air purifiers being used in antenatal clinics, hospitals, doctors' surgeries, and indeed anywhere that the public meet and where germs and infections are readily passed from one person to another via the atmosphere.

Stretch marks

As the breasts and stomach grow bigger, the skin stretches phenomenally, and unfortunately this can lead to permanent stretch marks – tiny scars in the underlying tissues of the skin. Once formed, these scars are very difficult to get rid of, and prevention is better than cure. A twice daily massage with a stomach massage oil (see page 115) will reduce the likelihood of stretch marks. All that is necessary is to gently rub the oil into the skin of the abdomen using sweeping movements. The massage itself will feel good, and I am sure the baby will like it, too. Anyone who already has stretch marks from a pregnancy or through losing weight quickly during dieting, need not

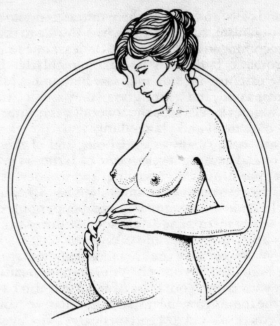

despair as a daily rub with the massage oil, will eventually bring about an improvement.

Taking good care of yourself

Water is very good for pregnant women – drinking lots of mineral water, swimming regularly and taking relaxing aromatic baths. For an aromatic bath, almost any essential oils that you particularly like will benefit you, and it is simply a matter of personal preference. **Clary sage** is a great morale booster, especially towards the end of pregnancy when each day seems like an eternity, and one wonders if the baby is ever going to arrive!

As mentioned earlier, **lavender** oil is very beneficial. It has the ability to stimulate the production of healthy white blood cells, and to goad them into action, should an invading organism, such as a cold virus, decide to drop in. I would recommend a lavender bath at least once a week. Other aromatic baths can be taken regularly. Light, refreshing essences include **melissa**, **bergamot**, **lemon**, **orange**, **rosewood**, and **lemongrass** – they are all citrousy. Heavier, sweeter smells are **sandalwood**, **geranium**, **rose**, **jasmine**, **patchouli** and **ylang-ylang**.

There are many, many essential oils, and of the most common ones, I have mentioned those of particular interest to me. **Peppermint** is very cooling, and wonderful for a cooling bath in the midst of summer. I was heavily pregnant during a heatwave one summer, and peppermint baths saved my sanity many times! Just add 2-4 drops to a bath of tepid water, mix well, slide in and relax.

During your pregnancy you are a most important person, and must take care of yourself. Your state of health will reflect on your baby. Your state of mind will also have an effect on the foetus growing inside you. Whatever you eat, whatever you drink and to a certain degree, whatever you apply to your skin, will be building blocks for the growth and formation of your child. We can help to grow beautiful babies, just as we grow beautiful flowers and plants, with careful nurturing and attention. It completely amazes me that the nine months needed to grow another human being, seems too long a time for some women to do without their favourite habit, even though it may be extremely harmful to the unborn child. But habits *are* sometimes hard to break and a safe alternative, such as clary sage baths to lift depression and thereby possibly reduce the consumption of alcohol, may be worth a try.

Also remember **Rescue Remedy**, which is extremely useful to take at times of stress. It can really calm you down, and anyone who instinctively reaches for a cigarette when under pressure or feeling upset, may find the ability to break with their smoking habit when they find that a glass of water to which Rescue Remedy has been added really does restore calmness.

Heartburn

The part of pregnancy I most hated and dreaded was the heartburn. I suffered with it for about six weeks, with each pregnancy. When expecting my first child, I took **peppermint** oil, which had helped enormously with the earlier nausea. It helped, but I can still remember waking up every two hours during the night, to take another drop, just so that I could go back to sleep again. When my second child was on the way, Robert suggested I take **rose** oil, and I found that this afforded me longer heartburn-relief than the peppermint. However, by the time I was expecting my third and last child, Robert had discovered, in some ancient text, that **sandalwood** was good for heartburn, as it was a bitter-tasting essential oil. I took one drop, and hated the taste, but it worked. One dose was all I needed to see me through the day. Another drop in the evening, and I slept soundly throughout the night. I could not tolerate anything sweet, and for this reason I did not take the **sandalwood** oil on sugar or in honey water, although this is normally the best method.

Although **sandalwood** oil is bitter tasting, it is not too unpleasant to take neat. I find the most convenient way to take it is a single drop on the tongue.

Constipation

Constipation during pregnancy is uncomfortable, unhealthy for both the mother and the baby, and usually unnecessary if a sensible pattern of eating is followed. I was already a vegetarian before any of my children were

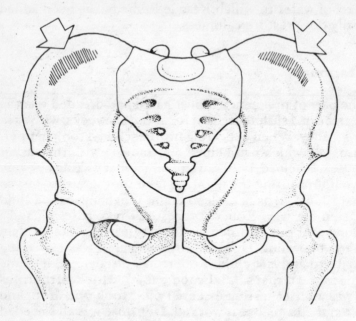

conceived, and although I would not expect everyone to follow suit, it does help to cut down the intake of heavy foods, such as meat and cheese; eat lots of fresh vegetables and fruit, drink plenty of mineral water, and replace white bread and rice with wholemeal bread and other whole grain foods, each day.

Because tension can be a contributing factor towards constipation, the relaxing baths are recommended.

For anyone who does suffer badly from constipation, I would recommend a massage of the lower back area using a simple blend of oils (see page 115). Pay particular attention to the area at either side of the spine, within the pelvic frame (see above). It is quite possible to do this massage to yourself whilst standing up, but do exert a little pressure and slide your fingertips in a circular motion.

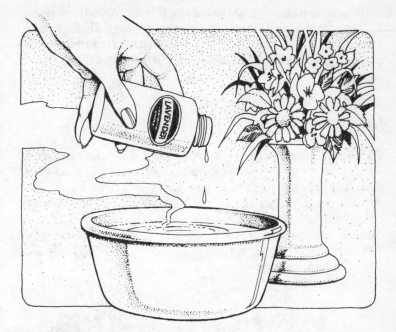

Purifying the atmosphere

It used to be standard practice for doctors and midwives to don white facial masks before delivering the baby, but I hope this relatively pointless ritual has now been abandoned. Airborne bacteria are so tiny that they penetrate through the gauze masks as soon as the wearer speaks or coughs, so there seems little point in them being worn, unless it is for the psychological benefit of the woman in labour. However, airborne bacteria are vulnerable to essential oil vapours so, whether giving birth at home or in hospital, keep a small bowl of warm water by the bedside, to which should be added **bergamot** or **lavender**. (See page 115). These, and many more essential oils are anti-bacterial agents, and their use will give you the satisfaction of knowing that, even if your midwife happens to have a cold, and even though the doctors' shoes are not sterile, you and your new baby have an extra measure of protection, invisible to the eye, but very perceptible to the nose.

Labour massage

Providing that you have a sympathetic partner or friend willing to sit with you during labour, you will find great comfort from a firm massage to your lower back. This should be done with the heel of the hand, in between contractions. As relaxation is of paramount importance (and I am assuming that the expectant mother is *not* sedated with drugs), a simple blend of essential oils (see

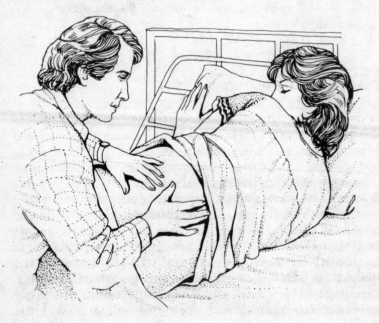

page 115) in a vegetable oil base, will help ease the pain in the muscles, and coupled with the firm pressure of the massage, the experience is very welcome. This massage need not be given continuously, especially if the labour is a particularly long one, but just now and again when the woman feels the need. My first labour was of twenty-seven hours duration and, as I was determined to 'do it naturally' without any drugs, but as the hours involved were long, I'm afraid that after the birth of our son, my husband was more in need of recuperation than I was! However, I do feel that, whenever it is humanly possible to give birth to a baby without resorting to the usual cocktail of hospital medications, the baby benefits, you benefit, and the bond between mother and baby is forged forever. The bliss of childbirth, the overwhelming love which pours forth to welcome the new human being is not hampered, and within minutes the pain and trauma of labour pales into insignificance.

Pain relief

A good deal of preparation for labour is advisable, and there are many books (see Further Reading) written about the appropriate exercises for the different groups of muscles. Regular practice of these exercises is an invaluable aid to happy labour, but there is one muscle which cannot be exercised in advance, and that is the muscle of the cervix (the neck of the womb). It is this muscle which has to stretch open to allow the passage of the baby's head, and this is obviously going to be a painful process, after all, it is that small but strong muscle which has sealed your baby within the womb for the past nine months. Well into my labour when I was beginning to fantasize about a general anaesthetic, my husband applied a hand-hot **clary sage*** compress to my lower abdomen, just above the pubic hair. The relief from pain was incredible, and I neither wanted nor needed anything else for the duration of labour. This compress can only be applied when the woman is lying down, and I know that many women prefer other positions. If the compress is used, it should be renewed as soon as it cools down and, as it is being changed frequently, it is not necessary to cover it with a dry cloth. An alternative to the compress, is a **clary sage** oil massage (see Chapter 9 page 115). During my pregnancies I also took homoeopathic *Caulophyllum*, to strengthen and tone the womb, and with each of my children's births the pushing stage lasted only five minutes.

For more information about homoeopathic remedies, see Further Reading.

*Calendula tincture (homoeopathic remedy) is equally effective.

7.
AFTER THE BIRTH

It amazes me that any woman should ever have died from post-partum infection. Yet many thousands have, over the years, due to our ignorance regarding hygiene.

Knowing of the antiseptic and protective powers of essential oils, I cannot help but wonder why childbirth is not always accompanied by pertinent use of essential oils.

As all essential oils, to a greater or lesser degree, have antiseptic properties and, when used in their correct diluted form, do not cause any problems or unwanted side effects, it makes sense to use them. Essential oils heal and protect the skin from bacteria, and a newly-delivered mother is indeed vulnerable to infection.

Healing the perineum

If you were unlucky enough to have had an episiotomy, or have torn, then the perineum will require gentle care to help it heal speedily and without too much discomfort. After giving birth to my children, getting to know them and putting them to the breast, the first thing I did for myself was have a sitz bath with **cypress** and **lavender** (see Chapter 9 page 115). Cypress is astringent and causes the raw blood vessels to close over, and lavender oil is very healing, and gently encourages the growth of new skin at

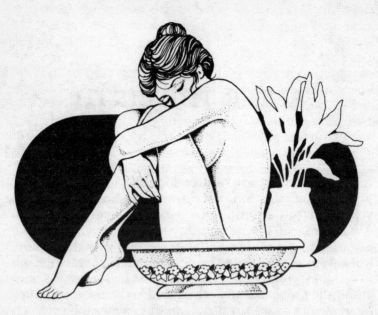

the same time as protecting the raw areas.

A new plastic bowl is ideal for a sitz bath. If you are small like me, then a washing-up bowl is adequate. For larger ladies a baby bath would be necessary. I would keep the bowl and essences in the bathroom, and have a sitz bath after every visit to the toilet. As the perineal skin heals up quickly, the stitches (if any have been needed) can be removed by the midwife a few days earlier, and this makes sitting a more pleasant experience.

Sore nipples

Prevention is better than cure, and a regime for preparing the nipples for the onslaught of a hungry baby is definitely advisable. I know of several women who, although desperate to breastfeed their babies, were unable to because of the pain and the bleeding. Even if the nipple does not bleed, many babies have quite a grip, and even the most prepared nipples can feel sore. Most essential oils are too strong for use on this sensitive area, and would also be inadvisable for the baby to swallow, not to mention the taste. However, sore nipples will benefit from applying a dilute **rose** (see page 116) and, although the nipple should be thoroughly washed before each feeding session, no harm will come to the baby should any be swallowed.

Post-natal depression

Post-natal depression usually arrives with the milk, on day three or four after the birth. It is due to a hormone adjustment in the body, and most women get weepy and miserable for a few days and then recover, but a few unfortunate women suffer for months and months, to such a degree that they cannot feel any love for their child. My experience of post-natal depression was that of falling from a euphoric high into a bottomless pit of misery, from whose depths I was not able to see a way out. I couldn't bear to talk to my husband and demanded a divorce (which is not the best thing to ask for when you have a three-day-old daughter!) Rather than acknowledge my request, he ran a bath for me, to which was first added a few drops of **jasmine**. I began to feel better almost as soon as I stepped into the bath and afterwards I went to sleep with a drop of **jasmine** oil on the edge of my pillow. When I woke up from my sleep, I was no longer suffering from post-natal depression. It had completely gone, and I was able to laugh at the way I had been just a few hours earlier.

If **jasmine** oil is not on hand, then **ylang-ylang** or **clary sage** oil are almost as effective.

Lactation problems

Usually a woman's breasts produce milk spontaneously after the birth and, as the baby suckles, a further supply is generated: a case of supply and demand. Occasionally, though, there is not enough milk to satisfy the baby's hunger. This could be due to an inadequate diet or depleted energies in the mother, possibly caused by a very exhausting labour, or perhaps there are other children also demanding mother's attention. Fear of being unable to breastfeed can also impair the flow of milk.

I experienced a few days when my milk yield was definitely low, and so I took **fennel** oil; two drops in honey water, repeated every two hours. This oil always works to increase the milk flow, and I have heard that fennel is fed to cows for that same reason.

Mastitis

Sore breasts can be really painful, and can even induce a fever. It used to be called 'milk fever', and was sometimes fatal. Mastitis means 'inflammation of the mammaries' – which are the breasts. It can occur when the breast is not completely emptied of milk, or when a milk duct in the nipple gets clogged. So it is important to express milk from whichever breast has a surplus, and also to wash the nipples carefully after every feed.

If mastitis should occur, then the most important thing is to reduce the heat in the local area. A compress of **lavender, geranium** and **rose** (see Chapter 9), will take away much of the heat and discomfort. If the temperature continues to rise or does not return to normal, consult a doctor.

If the symptoms should come on during the night and you decide to wait until morning before calling in the doctor, then the following can be employed. A **eucalyptus** foot bath, together with the breast compress, will bring down the temperature temporarily, and this could be repeated every two hours. You should otherwise remain in bed, but do not allow yourself to get overheated with too many bedclothes. The breast compress should be freshly applied every hour or so, and the nipple washed before breast feeding. If you feel strong enough, then have a **lavender** bath, with just comfortably warm water, and get someone to help you in and out of the bath.

Mastitis also occurs when breast feeding is stopped abruptly, in which case the same treatment would apply.

Tiredness

Labour can be intensely tiring but, with adequate rest and nutritious meals, one's strength should soon return. However, babies have a habit of being rather inconsiderate of their mother's requirements and often cause havoc with the night's sleep. Acute tiredness can be remedied with morning **rosemary** baths, and taking a nap whenever possible. But for chronic tiredness and lack of energy, I would recommend that advice be sought from an acupuncturist or Mc Timony chiropractor (see Useful Addresses).

It is now, after the birth, that a woman deserves and needs, more than at any other time, a good massage. Labour is physically very demanding, and can take a lot out of you, but a back and leg massage with a blend of essential oils of your choice, will give renewed energy and strength. For an energizing back massage oil see page 111.

8.

REMEDIES FOR CHILDHOOD ILLNESSES

In this chapter I will use case histories from a variety of illnesses my own children have experienced. As long as they are available, I feel that I may as well make use of doctors, in the way of diagnosis, and occasionally refer to them when I am confounded. However, I have so far never accepted a prescription for medications, instead preferring to use *essential oils* and *homoeopathic remedies* whenever possible. My children presently range from five to ten years of age and up to now not one of them has even been given a 'junior' aspirin.

I do not suggest that parents should abandon their doctors, and start to treat serious illnesses by themselves, but I include this chapter for those parents who, like me, feel that course after course of antibiotics cannot be beneficial for a child and very much prefer to treat their children 'holistically'. I do recognize that antibiotics, those 'magic bullets' invented in the early twentieth century, have their uses, and I was grateful for their existence on one occasion when I was very ill, but that was the only time I have used them in a span of twelve years.

Every ailment described in this chapter is one I have either nursed my own children through, or advised a friend coping with a sick child. I know that essential oils work, and often they are all that is required, but I would like to point out that a knowledge of homoeopathy is a very valuable aid to any mother of young children.

I always keep a wide selection of homoeopathic remedies, essential oils and Bach Flower remedies at home. Over the years I have become quite expert in successfully treating myself and my family. However, correct diagnosis is important and, if seriously in doubt, then you should always consult your doctor, or seek the help of a homoeopath.

You are the best nurse

You are the best nurse your child could ever have. You have the love that your child needs, and the security of being at home with the family is very important to a sick child. All you need is the confidence and knowledge to treat children's illnesses with the correct remedy, coupled with infinite amounts of patience.

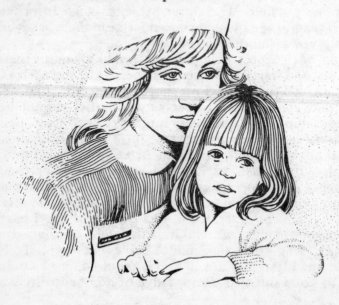

My feeling is that children are vibrant, healthy beings and, given the right help and support during an acute attack of some virus or other, their own body's defence mechanism will spring into action, and cope very efficiently with the invading organism, whatever it may be. I cannot see the necessity in prescribing antibiotics for little children every time they succumb to an illness. Antibiotics are wonderful when used in very severe cases, and can be lifesavers, but when routinely given for acute illnesses which would respond just as quickly to gentler natural remedies, they can be indiscriminate cell destroyers, and if over-used could bring about a decline in the health of the child. Everything has its place, so let us keep antibiotics in their place – in reserve, for the time when a powerful drug is really called for.

Dry skin in newborn infants

My son had dry, wrinkled skin when he was born, and looked like a beautiful but tiny 'old man'. I did not want to use a mineral-based baby oil from a chemist (mineral oil is fine for preventing nappy rash, but not for treating dry skin) and instead gently rubbed the dry areas with a **sweet almond** oil and **rose** blend. (See page 117).

Babies' skin is very delicate, and I do not advise the use of essential oils, except for a minute amount of **rose** oil in a base oil. After bathing the baby and drying gently, rub in a little dilute **rose** oil. I found this preferable to creams and powders, and the added bonus is that your baby smells even lovelier.

Colic

It is one thing to be woken up three times a night to feed

and change your baby, but something else altogether when he starts screaming at about seven o'clock in the evening and continues well into the night. Nothing you do comforts him, and the only recourse is to pace the floor until the infant drops off to sleep again. Colic seems to stay with a baby for several months after the first attack. Having found that a dose of proprietory gripe water did not cure the condition, but merely quietened the crying for up to an hour, I decided that I was not prepared to have my new baby swallowing the quantities of sugar that gripe water contains and decided upon a compress. **Camomile*** oil was chosen for its soothing qualities, and one drop was added to a bowl of warm water. After mixing thoroughly, a handkerchief was wrung out in the **camomile** water, and applied to the baby's tummy. Then a small dry towel was placed on top. This only needs to be left on for about half an hour, or until the baby drops off to sleep. Take care to keep the baby warm when the compress is on the abdomen.

Never be tempted to use more essential oil in the hope that it will work better or quicker. It will not. A baby's skin is very delicate, and this must always be respected.

---

*Camomile is quite an expensive oil, and although I have found it to be unsurpassed, the next best oil would be **geranium**, applied in the same manner.

Heat bumps

Babies can quickly get overheated during hot weather, and their way of letting mother know is to cry. Often the face has little red bumps on it. The child should be undressed and allowed to cool down. A lukewarm bath, to which one drop of **lavender** has been added, is both cooling and calming.

Nosebleeds

When young children have a nose bleed, they usually become very frightened and even hysterical at the sight of their own blood. Adult remedies, such as putting a bunch of keys down the back, are not really appropriate. Again, **lavender** will help. Put one or two drops of **lavender** or **cypress** into a small bowl of cold water, wring out a handkerchief in the liquid, and lay it over the bridge of the nose. The bleeding should stop very quickly and, because of the soothing properties of **lavender**, the child will soon be calmed.

Toothache

If children are not given too many sweet things to eat, then the likelihood of toothache is remote. But there may be an occasion when a tooth aches, and perhaps there is a day or so to wait before a visit to a dentist can be arranged. For an older child, a drop of **clove** or **peppermint** oil on a small piece of cotton wool, and placed on the affected tooth, will take away some of the pain. Because of the strong taste this is probably not suitable for a young child, and in this instance a **lavender** compress would be more acceptable. Put one drop of **lavender** in warm water, then apply the wet cloth to the face over the ache and keep warm.

Teething babies will stop crying and go to sleep when a drop of **lavender** or **camomile** oil is placed on the edge of their pillow. Also putting a drop on a piece of their clothing, so that they inhale the vapours, will calm down a fractious child.

Earache

Earache was, for me, a distressing part of my childhood. I

seemed to have recurrent bouts of it, and was given salt packs, cotton wool soaked in castor oil, and aspirin. None of these seemed to work very well, and I wish that my mother had known about **lavender**. One drop on a small piece of cotton wool and placed *gently* in the outer ear, will work wonders. The healing vapours find their way into the inner ear and take away the pain.

Colds and stuffiness

At the first signs of a cold in any of my children, I put them to bed with a drop of **eucalyptus** oil on each side of the pillow. Sometimes this treatment alone is sufficient to stop the cold from progressing. Common sense should also prevail in the treatment of colds and, as milk and dairy products are known to be 'mucus producing', it is sensible to eliminate these from the diet until the cold has gone.

Tetchiness/tantrums

If children do not have a sound night's sleep, they can be pretty hard to handle the following morning. On occasions, one of my children wakes up in a 'don't want to eat any breakfast/get dressed/go to school' mood and, better than reasoning, I have found the simplest thing to do is put that child in a **clary sage** bath, and leave for ten minutes. The difference in attitude is amazing, quite a transformation. Every time I have used a **clary sage** bath for a grumpy child the moodiness has completely vanished within minutes and the child gets out smiling and ready for the day.

Fever – general

When the body temperature rises above normal, whether

due to a cold, flu or one of the common childhood illnesses, it sometimes becomes impossible for the child to sleep.

It is common practice for junior aspirin to be given to children sporting a fever, but I prefer instead to gently but quickly bathe my child in a lukewarm **lavender** bath (three-four drops). On the occasions when I have used this treatment, even when all other soothing fails, the lavender bath soothes, cools and calms the child, and allows him or her to fall asleep again. If a child's temperature reaches very high levels (103°F/39°C) a doctor should always be consulted, but I have found that lower temperatures can be controlled with the prudent use of essential oils. Once, when my son – then one year old – had a high temperature, I wrapped his feet in **eucalyptus** compresses (two drops **eucalyptus** in a bowl of cold water), and renewed with a fresh one as soon as the cloth felt warm. In this way I was able to nurse him from a dangerously high fever back to a safe level in a short time and without the need for aspirin suppositories. Children can go into convulsions if their temperature soars too high, and therefore to actively work towards normalizing the body heat is much less stressful to parents than watching helplessly as the temperature goes up and up.

Chicken pox

To help a child throw off the chicken pox virus, I would not hesitate to recommend that he or she be given a homoeopathic remedy just as soon as the virus has manifested itself on the skin (see Further Reading). Prompt treatment can, and does, clear up chicken pox in under one week. However, there is still the problem of itching, and it is difficult to stop a child from scratching. This can lead to permanent damage to the skin, in the form of 'pock marks'.

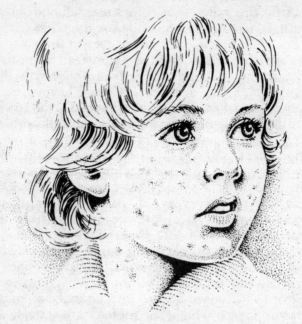

As each of my children went down with chicken pox (thankfully *not* simultaneously), I dosed them with the homoeopathic remedy, and dabbed their skin with **peppermint** lotion. Knowing that **peppermint** oil was cooling and soothing, but not wishing to put my spotty youngsters into a bath, I made up a lotion to apply externally to the skin.

To a 1 litre (1¾ pint) bottle of water I added *one* drop of **peppermint** oil, and then shook the bottle vigorously. I then poured away half the contents, topped up with water, and shook the bottle again. I then repeated these steps, and so had *¼ drop* of **peppermint** oil in *1 litre (1¾ pints)* of water. I applied this to the spots, using cotton wool. My son immediately noticed the difference, and did not feel the need to scratch any more. I subsequently used this lotion on my two daughters, with similarly good results. Shingles in adults, will also benefit from this treatment, but add a drop of **geranium** to the bottle of water.

Croup/whooping cough

These respiratory diseases are very frightening to both the child and its parents because of the constriction of the airways. Steam vapours in the sick room will help the child to breathe more freely. The addition of essences to the hot water will greatly enhance the treatment, especially if the chosen essential oil has anti-spasmodic properties. Essences which fall into this category are **basil, clary sage, cypress, eucalyptus, hyssop, juniper, lavender,** and **rosemary**. Any one of these essences (one or two drops) is sufficient to make the atmosphere beneficial to the sick child. A compress of either **lavender** or **cypress** oil laid on the chest will aid in the recovery from the virus. The chest compress should be made up using warm water, and covered with a dry fluffy towel. As soon as the compress starts to cool it should be removed or replaced with a fresh, warm compress.

In tending to a very sick child oneself there is less opportunity for you, the parent, to become distressed, and a calm mother will help the child to remain calm, which is important when treating spasmodic disorders.

Asthma

Asthma in children is something I have never had dealings with, although I was told by doctors that my son with eczema would inevitably develop asthma. He never did, and I believe that was because I would not allow the use of steroids or coal tar preparations on his skin. These creams and ointments do make the eczema disappear and leave the skin smooth, but they do not remove the underlying allergy that causes both the eczema and the asthma. At the risk of upsetting many orthodox opinions, I would urge parents to seek the help of a good homoeopath, and and not to allow the use of skin steroids or any preparation which is going to suppress the disease.

Aching legs

When your child wakes in the night, crying and moaning about 'achy legs' it is no comfort to be told that it is 'just growing pains'. Usually the calf muscles are sore or in spasm. I am not sure why it happens to some children and not others, but two of my three children have been affected in this way, and the entire household has been woken in the night by the distress caused. I give the child a homoeopathic remedy (see Further Reading) and massage the legs

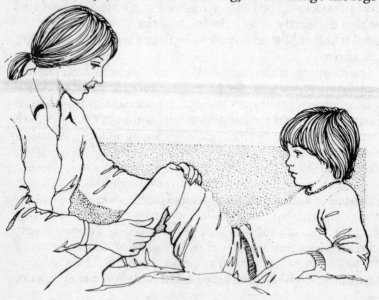

from ankle to knee with a simple blend of essences (see page 117) in vegetable oil, which I keep for such emergencies. Usually we can all go back to sleep within fifteen minutes.

Stomach ache

My children often get a 'tummy ache' after having attended a birthday party, because everything that is sweet and gooey and normally rationed is available in vast quantities, and what child can resist? It is normally on getting into bed that my children complain of pains, and after giving them a dose of **peppermint** oil (one drop in a glass of honey water) all is usually well. For more severe spasms, a **camomile** compress to the lower abdomen always works. (See page 117).

Convulsions

A doctor should always be called if a child goes into convulsions, but whilst you are waiting for your doctor to arrive there are certain things you can do. Remove all clothing and place the child into a lukewarm **lavender** bath, supporting the head with one hand and gently wetting the child's body with the other. Just a few minutes is long enough, then wrap the child in a large bath towel, to prevent him getting chilled. As a convulsing child is a frightening sight, I recommend that the parents should take a dose of Rescue Remedy to allay their panic.

Headache (severe)

Children do not get severe headaches unless they are very

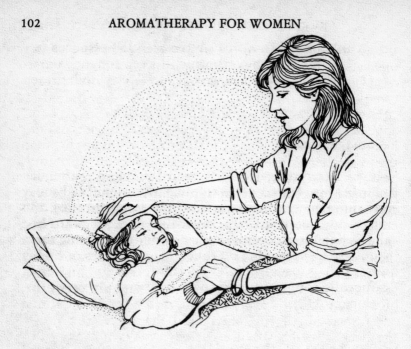

ill (such as with meningitis) or have sunstroke or concussion from a fall. Therefore a doctor should be consulted immediately.

However, while waiting for the doctor to arrive, a homoeopathic remedy can be administered, which will not interfere with conventional treatment, and a **geranium** compress can be applied to the forehead to relieve anxiety, and reduce pain. This treatment was most satisfactory when we were waiting for a doctor to come and examine Saffron, then four years old, for suspected meningitis.

Head lice

If you have school or playgroup age children, you will undoubtedly have encountered the dreaded head lice.

When my children were infected (and one-for-all, all-for-one seems to be the head lice motto) I decided to try a treatment with essential oils recommended by Robert (see page 114).

I sectioned the hair from the forehead to the neck, and applied the 'lice mixture' to the scalp, until the roots of the hair were saturated. Then a little more oil was applied to the remainder of the hair. I then piled the hair on top of the head (in the case of the girls, who have long hair) and wrapped a long sheet of cling-film tightly around the head, and behind the ears. I was not sure how my children would endure this treatment but they loved it, and scampered about being 'space-invaders' for a couple of hours! When the cling-film was removed, over the bath, most of the 'problem' went with it. The next step was a good hair-wash. As with all oily hair treatments, shampoo needs to be applied first, to make an emulsion, and then water. After washing thoroughly I used the regulation fine-toothed 'nit comb', to dislodge any eggs which may still have adhered to the hair strands. I repeated this treatment after three days, and not only were my children completely lice-free, but they were the owners of lustrous, shining, healthy hair. All the schools in that area of the country had problems with lice infestation, and one of my friends bought a proprietory bottle of lice-killer from her chemists. She reported to me later that it had irritated her son's head and his hair had started falling out. It had also been necessary to keep him away from school for forty-eight hours whilst the foul-smelling treatment dried naturally and did its job.

Eczema

I do not recommend that essential oils be used in cases of infantile eczema, as the skin is so sensitive, and delicate.

In my experience, infantile eczema responds well to homoeopathic treatment, but expert advice should be sought. There are two proprietary creams which I recommend to soothe the itching, one is Nelson's Calendula Cream and the other is Rescue Remedy.

Pre-party nerves

Adults are not the only ones to suffer from pre-party nerves and, with children, the eagerly anticipated party suddenly produces floods of tears and pleas to stay at home. If either of my daughters became keyed up before a party, I would pop her into a **geranium** bath (two drops only) as it always relaxed them and relieved anxiety. Making a perfume for

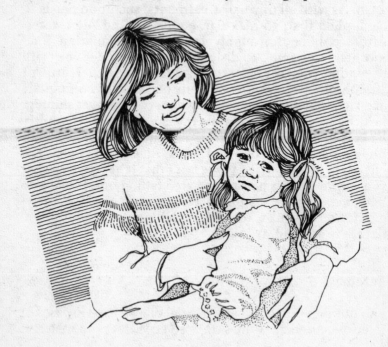

a little girl is relatively simple (see page 117). The blend, which will depend upon the character of your child, will be unique to her.

9.
RECIPES

Recipes for Chapter 1

Muscular aches (massage oil)
10 drops **juniper**
7 drops **lavender**
8 drops **rosemary**

in 2 fl oz (50ml) vegetable oil

Hangover (bath)
2 drops **fennel**
2 drops **juniper**
2 drops **rosemary**

Recipes for Chapter 2

Period pains (massage oil)
15 drops **clary sage**

in 2 fl oz (50ml) vegetable oil

Herpes (massage oil) for applying to the glands at the top inside leg
8 drops **rose**
17 drops **lavender**

in 2 fl oz (50ml) vegetable oil

Thrush (douche)
2   drops rose
4   drops lavender
2   drops bergamot

in 2 pints (1 litre) warm water. Shake well in a bottle. Add to douche/enema pot.

Pruritus (sitz bath)
1   drop rose
1   drop peppermint

in large bowl of warm water

Leucorrhea (douche)
as for thrush

Cystitis (lotion)
1   drop lavender

in 3 fl oz (100ml) water. If a smallish plastic bottle is used, it could be taken to work. But the mixture will need to be discarded and a fresh one made up every *third* day.

Recipes for Chapter 3

Breast developer (massage oil)
9   drops geranium
16 drops ylang-ylang

in 2 fl oz (50ml) vegetable oil

Thigh slimmer (massage oil)
13 drops cypress
12 drops juniper

in 2 fl oz (50ml) vegetable oil

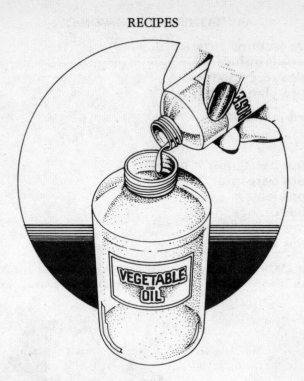

Aphrodisiac massage oil
5 drops **jasmine**
5 drops **rose**
10 drops **sandalwood**
5 drops **bergamot**

in 2 fl oz (50ml) vegetable oil

A **rose** *perfume*
4 drops **rose**
12 drops **sandalwood**
2 drops **geranium**
2 drops **rosewood**

in 10ml jojoba

A heady, **jasmine** *perfume*
2   drops **jasmine**
12 drops **rosewood**
6   drops **ylang-ylang**

in 10ml jojoba

eau de Cologne
20 drops **petitgrain** *or* **neroli**
80 drops **bergamot**
30 drops **lemon**
40 drops **orange**
20 drops **lavender**
10 drops **rosemary**

add to 100ml for 10 per cent dilution (200ml for 5 per cent dilution) distilled (or mineral) water and shake.

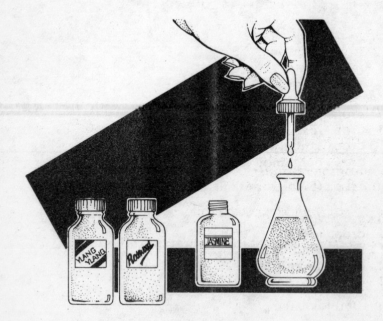

Bedroom to boudoir
Lashings of exotic essences (e.g. **jasmine, rose, patchouli, sandalwood, ylang-ylang**). Imagination.

Recipes for Chapter 4

Mouthwash
1 drop **peppermint** or **fennel**
1 drop **lemon**

in ½ pint (285ml) water

Resistance builder (massage oil)
20 drops **lavender**
5 drops **bergamot**

in 2 fl oz (50ml) vegetable oil

Invigorating massage oil
17 drops **rosewood**
6 drops **orange**
2 drops **geranium**

in 2 fl oz (50ml) vegetable oil

Relaxing massage oil
13 drops **lavender**
2 drops **geranium**
10 drops **sandalwood**

in 2 fl oz (50ml) vegetable oil

Shingles (**peppermint** lotion) (**geranium** lotion)
as for chicken pox (page 117)

Depression (pick-me-up bath)
2 drops **clary sage**
2 drops **bergamot**
2 drops **ylang-ylang**

add to bath water; mix well.

Recipes for Chapter 5: skin care

Oil for dry skin
10 drops **sandalwood**
7 drops **geranium**
3 drops **rosewood**
5 drops **ylang-ylang**

in 2 fl oz (50ml) vegetable oil

Oil for acne/oily skin
12 drops **cypress**
13 drops **lemon**

in 2 fl oz (50ml) vegetable oil

Oil for mature skin
8   drops **frankincense** or **myrrh**
14 drops **lavender**
3   drops **neroli**

in 2 fl oz (50ml) vegetable oil

Skin tonics – floral waters

Normal/dry skin
4 drops **geranium**
6 drops **lavender**

in 2 fl oz (50ml) water (preferably bottled spring water)

Greasy skin
6   drops **bergamot**
4   drops **lavender**

in 2 fl oz (50ml) water (preferably bottled spring water)

Rose *body rub*
20 drops **rose**
5ml jojoba

in 2 fl oz (50ml) almond oil

Facial mask
1 heaped tablespoon kaolin or Fuller's earth powder
2 tablespoons water
½ teaspoon clear honey
1   drop **lavender**
1   drop **geranium**

Neroli *compress*
1   drop **neroli**

in bowl of warm water (approx. 1 pint/570ml). Soak a flannel or strips of towelling in liquid. Squeeze out excess, and lay the compress over your face. (Ideally the cloth should have a hole cut out for your nose.)

Recipes for Chapter 5: hair care

Treatment for greasy hair
12 drops **bergamot**
13 drops **lavender**
5   ml jojoba

in 2 fl oz (50ml) vegetable oil

Treatment for dandruff
10 drops **eucalyptus**
15 drops **rosemary**
5 ml jojoba

in 2 fl oz (50ml) vegetable oil

Treatment for hair damaged by bleaching/perming
15 drops **rosewood**
5 drops **geranium**
5 drops **sandalwood**
5 drops **lavender**
10 ml jojoba

in 2 fl oz (50ml) vegetable oil

Treatment for head lice
25 drops **rosemary**
12 drops **eucalyptus**
13 drops **geranium**
25 drops **lavender**

in 3 fl oz (75ml) vegetable oil

Hair rinses

dark hair
3 drops **rosemary**
1 drop **rosewood**
1 drop **geranium**

in 2 pints (1 litre) water

fair hair
2 drops **camomile**
1 drop **lemon**

to a 2 pint (1 litre) bottle of water, add the drops of essence.
Cap and shake well. Essential oils do not dissolve in water,
but shaking vigorously will disperse them sufficiently.

Shake again, prior to pouring over the hair. If you have short hair you will not need to use 1 litre of hair rinse, and the mixture may safely be kept for a few days, until your next shampoo.

Recipes for Chapter 6

Stretch marks (massage oil)
20 drops **lavender**
5   drops (optional) **neroli**

in 2 fl oz (50ml) wheatgerm oil

Constipation (massage oil)
20 drops **marjoram**
5   drops **rose**

in 2 fl oz (50ml) vegetable oil

Labour (massage oil)
14 drops **clary sage**
5   drops **rose**
6   drops **ylang ylang**

in 2 fl oz (50 ml) vegetable oil

Antiseptic (room freshener)
6   drops **bergamot** or **lavender**

in a bowl: approx 1 pint (570ml) water

Recipes for Chapter 7

Healing the perineum (sitz bath)
2   drops **cypress**
3   drops **lavender**

in a large bowl of water, or shallow bath.

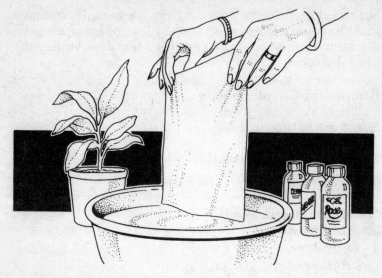

Mastitis (compress)
1   drop **geranium**
1   drop **lavender**
2   drops **rose**

in 1½ pints (850ml) cold water

Sore nipples (massage oil)
1   drop **rose**

in ¾fl oz (20ml) sweet almond oil

Recipes for Chapter 8

Head lice (massage oil)
25 drops **rosemary**
12 drops **eucalyptus**
13 drops **geranium**
25 drops **lavender**

in 3 fl oz (100ml) vegetable oil

Chicken pox (lotion)
1   drop **peppermint**

in 2 pint (1 litre) bottle of water

Add drop to water, cap and shake. Pour off half the
contents. Refill with water. Cap and shake. Pour away half
the contents. Refill with water. You are now left with ¼
drop oil to 2 pints (1 litre) water.

Aching legs (massage oil)
15 drops **lavender**
10 drops **rosemary**

in 2 fl oz (50ml) vegetable oil

Tummy ache (compress)
1   drop **camomile**

in 1 litre warm water (mix thoroughly).

Dry skin in infants (massage oil)
1   drop **rose**

in 2 fl oz (50ml) sweet almond oil

Children's bath
1   drop **geranium**
1   drop **orange**

mixed well in warm bath water.

Child's perfume
1   drop **geranium**
1   drop **orange**

in 5ml jojoba oil

Some useful conversions
1ml = 20 drops
5ml = 1 teaspoonful

GLOSSARY OF METHODS OF TREATMENT

Air Freshener

The essential oils of your choice added to a small bowl of warm water or the essences may be sprinkled on to the carpet, or placed on a radiator.

Compress

A piece of material soaked in water to which you have first added an essential oil. It will vary in size according to the area to be treated. A handkerchief is the correct size for a forehead compress for a headache; a cotton wool ball for an eye compress; a hand towel or face flannel for a stomach compress, etc. The water may be either warm or cold, again depending on what you are treating.

Sitz Bath

Also known as a hip bath. A few inches of water in the bottom of an ordinary bath, or a plastic bowl kept specially for this purpose. Add the selected essences and mix well in the water before sitting down.

Douche

An enema pot or plastic douche, both available from chemists, is filled with warm water and essences, which should first be thoroughly mixed together. Used in the treatment of vaginal disorders.

Honey Water

The easiest way of taking oils internally. Put one teaspoon of honey into a glass or cup, add 1 fl oz (30ml) of hot water and stir until honey is dissolved. Then add the drop or drops of essential oil.

Inhalation

Steam vapour inhalations consist of a bowl of hot water to which about 10 drops of essential oil are added. The purpose is to inhale the vapours.

Massage Oil

A blend of essential oils in a vegetable oil base, for a specific massage. The usual quantity is 2 per cent of essential oil plus 98 per cent vegetable oil, i.e. 40 drops of essential oil in 100ml of vegetable oil.

On A Pillow

When essential oils are used on a pillow, as in the case of **eucalyptus** for colds, the essence should be at the pillow's edge, and not come into contact with skin. To avoid staining the bed linen, only use the essences which are clear or light in colour.

Skin Rub Perfume

A delicately scented oil which can be rubbed into the entire body surface after bathing.

FURTHER READING

Aromatherapy

The Art of Aromatherapy by Robert Tisserand (C. W. Daniel, 1977).
The Practice of Aromatherapy by Dr Jean Valnet (C. W. Daniel, 1982).
Practical Aromatherapy by Shirley Price (Thorsons,1983).
Aromatherapy by Lautié and Passebecq (Thorsons 1984).

Homoeopathy

Homoeopathy: An Introductory Guide by Gordon Ross (Thorsons, 1976).
Homoeopathy: A Patient's Guide by Dr Anne Clover (Thorsons, 1984).
A Physician's Posy by Dr Dorothy Shepherd (Health Science Press, 1969).

Bach Flower Remedies

Bach Flower Therapy by Mechthild Scheffer (Thorsons, 1986).

Diet

Diet for a Small Planet by Frances Moore Lappé (Ballantine Books, 1975).

Vitamins

Thorsons Complete Guide to Vitamins and Minerals by Leonard Mervyn BSc. PhD, C.Chem, FRSC (Thorsons, 1986)
The Vitamin Bible by Earl Mindell (Arlington Books, 1979).

Childbirth

The Experience of Childbirth by Sheila Kitzinger (Penguin, 1979).
The Childbirth Book by Sheila Kitzinger (Fontana, 1980).

Reflexology

The Complete Guide to Foot Reflexology by Kevin and Barbara Kunz (Thorsons, 1984).
Reflexology: A Patient's Guide by Nicola M. Hall (Thorsons, 1986).

USEFUL ADDRESSES

The British Acupuncture Association
34 Alderney St
London SW1V 4EU

McTimony Chiropractic
The Institute of Pure Chiropractic
P.O. Box 127
Oxford
OX1 1HH

The British Homoeopathic Association
27a Devonshire Street
London W1N 1RJ

Dr Edward Bach Centre
Mount Vernon
Sotwell
Wallingford
Oxon

Essential Oils Suppliers

Many independent health food stores, and also the quality
health food chain stores, stock pure essential oils.

Essential oils may be obtained by post, by writing to:
Aroma-Therapy Supplies,
Unit W3, The Knoll Business Centre,
Old Shoreham Road,
Hove, Sussex BN3 7GS
(Tel: 0273 412139)

Also write to Aroma-Therapy Supplies for details of aromatherapy courses, seminars, your nearest stockist of essential oils, and for the address of your local aromatherapist.

Oils for aromatherapy have to be high quality *pure* essential oils, and not synthetic blends, so do make sure you buy from a reputable supplier.

INDEX

acne, oil for, 112
    treatment of, 66-7
air, to freshen, 18, 19, 115, 119
alcohol, 18, 41, 46
anaphrodisiacs, 36
antibiotics, 91, 93
aphrodisiacs, 35-6
    massage oil, 109
aromatic baths for relaxation, 22-3
asthma, 99
athlete's foot, 56

Bach flower remedies, 18, 48
basil oil, 14, 57, 61, 99
bergamot oil, 19, 26, 32, 33, 37, 53, 61, 76, 78, 81
blood-pressure, high, 59
body rubs, 70, 121
breasts, to enlarge, 39
    massage oil for, 108
burns, 55

camomile oil, 31, 71, 94, 95, 101
camphor oil, 53, 57, 60
cellulite, 40
chicken pox, 97
    lotion for, 117
clary sage oil, 18, 19, 26 29, 30, 36, 37, 51, 52, 61, 77, 83, 84, 87, 96, 99
clove oil, 58, 95
colds and stuffiness, 60, 96
compress, 119
conditioner, normal hair, 73
confidence, oil to boost, 37-8
constipation, 79, 80
    massage oil for, 115
convulsions, 101
croup, 99
cypress oil, 56, 58, 85, 95, 99
cystitis, 31
    lotion for, 108

dairy products, 46
dandruff, 73, 114
depression, 51
    aromatic bath for, 112
    post-natal, 87

diarrhoea, 19
diet, general, 46
distillation, 10
douching, vaginal, 32, 120
dry skin, 68
    in newborn infants, 93
    oils for, 112, 117

earache, 95-6
eau de Cologne, 110
eczema, 103-4
episiotomy, 85
essential oils, 10, 64-5, 66
eucalyptus oil, 32, 53, 60, 89, 96, 97, 99
exercise, importance of, 47
eye compresses, 70

facial masks, 69, 113
fainting, 57
feet, aching, 21
fennel oil, 26, 61, 88
fever, 96-7
fibre, 46
flatulence, 58
floral waters, 69
    greasy skin, 113
    normal/dry skin, 112
food allergies, 46
foot baths, 55
foot odour, 56
frankincense, 37, 68

geranium oil, 19, 23, 27, 37, 39, 61, 76, 88, 94, 102, 104

haemorrhoids (piles), 58
hair, damaged, treatment of, 71-2, 114
    greasy, treatment of, 72, 113
    rinses, dark and fair, 71, 114
hangover, 26
    remedy for, 107
head lice, 73, 102-3, 114, 116
headache, 57, 101-2
heartburn, 79
heat bumps, 94
herpes, genital, 32
    massage oil for, 107

homoeopathic remedies, 91
honey water, 120
hyssop, 99

indigestion, 58
influenza, 59
inhalation, 120
insomnia, 23-4

jasmine oil, 36, 38, 43, 51, 78, 87
jet lag, 17
jojoba oil, 41, 71
juniper oil, 30, 31, 40, 52, 99
labour, massage oil for, 115
    pain relief during, 83-4
lactation problems, 88
laryngitis, 59
lavender oil, 16, 17, 22, 23, 24, 25, 27, 31,
    32, 33, 53, 54, 55, 56, 57, 58, 60, 61, 68,
    76, 77, 81, 85, 88, 89, 94, 95, 96, 97, 99,
    101
legs, aching, 100
    massage oil for, 117
lemon oil, 19, 38, 61, 78
lemongrass oil, 18, 23, 30, 78
leucorrhoea, 33
    douche for, 108
linden blossom oil, 25, 39, 43, 76

marjoram oil, 25, 37, 59
massage, during labour, 82-3
    for muscular aches, 20-1
    importance of, 48-51
massage oil, 120
    invigorating, 111
    relaxing, 111
mastitis, 88
    compress for, 116
mature skin, 68
    oil for, 112
melissa oil, 19, 78
mental fatigue, 14
mouth wash, 61, 111
muscular aches, 20
    massage oil for, 107
myrrh oil, 68

nausea, during pregnancy, 75
Nelson's Calendular Cream, 104
neroli oil, 19, 23, 24, 25, 58, 68
    compress, 113
nerves, 104
nipples, sore, 86
    massage oil for, 116
nosebleeds, 95

olfaction, 40

orange oil, 37, 38, 78

party atmosphere, oils to induce, 37
patchouli oil, 36, 37, 39, 43, 78
peppermint oil, 16, 21, 26, 54, 57, 59, 61,
    75, 78, 95, 98, 101
perfume, child's, 117
    jasmine, 110
    rose, 109
    synthetic, 41
perineum, sitz bath to heal, 115
period pains, 29
    massage oil for, 107
premenstrual tension, 30
pruritus, 32
    sitz bath for, 108

Rescue Remedy, 18, 78, 101, 104
resistance builder (massage oil), 111
rose oil, 26, 32, 33, 36, 37, 39, 42, 61, 68,
    76, 88, 93
    body rub, 113
rosemary oil, 13, 18, 22, 26, 57, 71, 89, 99
rosewood oil, 19, 26, 37, 53, 78

sandalwood oil, 31, 36, 37, 43, 59, 60, 78,
    79
shingles, 61, 111
sitz bath, 119
slimming, oils to help, 52
spots, causes of, 53
    remedies for, 53
steroids, 99, 100
stomach ache, 101
stretch marks, 76
    massage oil for, 115
sunburn, 54
sweet almond oil, 93

tantrums, in children, 96
thighs, to slim, 39-40
    massage oil for, 108
throat, sore, 59
thrush (candida albicans), 31
    remedy for, 108
toothache, 58, 95
travel sickness, 16

ulcers, mouth, 53

vaginal discharge, 33
verruca, 57

water retention, 30
wheat germ oil, 65
whooping cough, 99

ylang-ylang oil, 17, 23, 30, 36, 37, 39, 43,
    51, 59, 61, 78, 87